Forage and
Grassland Management

Author

Professor (Dr) N. K. Prasad is a former Professor (Agronomy), BAU, Ranchi and Professor (Agriculture) in Ethiopian Universities is the recipient of the Common Wealth countries fellowship sponsored by the Reading University, UK for Post Doctoral Research and Training on "Micronutrients nutrition to a series of legumes" at CSIRO, QLD, Australia for his out-standing research achievement on Lucerne production in acid soils. of India. He is also the recipient of 'The "Best Paper Award" of the Indian Society of Agronomy, New Delhi. He has published about 100 research papers in different National and International Journals and guided several M.Sc. students in India and abroad encluding Ph.D. Scholars of Agronomy and Soil Sciences in India. Forage and Grassland Management is the third book to his credit after first one on "Soil Fertility and Plant Nutrition" and second one on "Stress Agronomy"

Forage and Grassland Management

–Author–
N.K. PRASAD

2014

Daya Publishing House®
A Division of
Astral International Pvt. Ltd.
New Delhi 110 002

Published by   :   **Daya Publishing House®**
A Division of
Astral International Pvt. Ltd.
– ISO 9001:2008 Certified Company –
4760-61/23, Ansari Road, Darya Ganj
New Delhi-110 002
Ph. 011-43549197, 23278134
E-mail: info@astralint.com
Website: www.astralint.com

Laser Typesetting   :   **Classic Computer Services**, Delhi - 110 035

Printed at   :   **Replika Press Pvt. Ltd.**

PRINTED IN INDIA

Preface

The sustainability of a farming system cannot be dreamed in absence of livestock vis-à-vis forage component without which the system is curtailed to only a cropping pattern. The drastic reduction in livestock population in general and draft animals in particular has virtually changed our Agriculture system to a susceptible enterprise. As such, intendive cropping system in absence of organic source of nutrients (manures) has virtually robbed the soils to such an extent that their productivity is declining day by day. The day is not very far off to result in crop failure similar to bouncing of cheque in absence of minimum balance desired in the account.

Though, we have achieved top position in total milk production in the world, even then, the per capita availability of milk in India is far from satisfactory. As such, we do not stand among 20 top countries in which availability of milk to per capita is more than India. Indigenous cows which are being reared on the farms as a by product may sustain on natural grasslands or the waste lands but it is very difficult to exploit the full milk production potential of cross- bred exotic cows on these resources. Since, high milking genotypes also needs adequate quantity of highly nutritious forages hence, sparing of some percentage (5-10%) of productive land to provide green vegetables (forages) is the need of the hour on the same pattern of putting productive land under vegetable cultivation for human consumption.. This will facilitate in bringing out stability in healthy livestock- soil- plant- human system. In addition to this, vital role of forage grasses and legumes as well as of non-palattble grasses in conserving soil, nutrients and moisture for a stable crop production in watersheds is also desired.

Therefore, keeping these mandates at hand, an attempt has been made to facilitate the proper management technology for growing forages and their components which may be an effective tool for Agricultural and animal husbandry teachers, students and to person's evolved in farming system.

The author acknowledges his gratitude to authors of different research papers and books from which possible help has been taken. The inspiration and encouragement received by Dr. A. P. Singh Professor (Forage Breeding) and Director Farm is duely acknowledged. My son Mr. Nrip Kishor Niraj also deserves special thanks for designing, photography and typing and as well as special thanks for my family members and friends for encouragement in preparing this book.

N.K. Prasad

Contents

Preface   v

List of Photographs and Figure   ix

List of Tables   xi

1. Introduction   1

2. Grasses and Legumes   9

3. Tropical Forage Cereals   17

4. Tropical Forage Grasses   31

5. Tropical Forage Legumes   57

6. Temperate Forage Crops   75

7. Temperate Forage Legumes   85

8. Forage Trees/Shrubs   97

9. Plant Population Dynamics   105

10. Grassland Distribution   109

11. Pasture Management   123

12. Range Management   133

13. Forage Preservation   141

14. Grass: Legume Associations   149

15. Nutrient Management   155

16. Agroforestry   167
17. Forages in Soil Conservation   173
    References   179
    Subject Index   187

List of Photographs and Figures

Photographs

1. Bajra (*Pennisetum glaucum* L.)
2. Teosinte (*Euchlena mexicana*)
3. Hybrid Napier (*Pennisetum perpureum*)
4. Thin Napier Grass / Mission Grass (*P. polystachyon* Sch.)
5. Sadabahar Grass / Gamba Grass (*Andropogan gayanus*)
6. Para Grass (*Brachiaria mutica*)
8. Guinea Grass (*Panicum maximum* Jacq.)
9. *Setaria sphaceolata*
10. Anjan grass (*Cenchrus ciliaris*)
11. Rhodes grass (*Chloris gayana* Kunth.)
12. Spear Grass (*Heteropogon contortus*)
14. Stylo (*Stylosanthes guinensis*)
15. Stylo (*Stylosanthes hamata*)
16. Stylo (*Stylosanthes humilis*)
17. Siratro (*Macroptilium atropurpureum*)
18. Centro (*Centrosema sps.*)
19. Kudzu vine (*Puraria thunbergia*)
20. Oats (*Avena sativa*)
21. Berseem / Egyptian Clover (*T. alexandrinum*)

22A. Lucerne/ Alfalfa/Rizka (*Medicago sativa L.*)
      Plant & Flower

22 B. Lucerne/ Alfalfa/Rizka (*Medicago sativa L.*) Flower,
      Pods and Seeds

23A. Subabul (*Leucaena leucocephala*)

23B. Subabul (*Leucaena leucocephala*) Pods & Seeds

24. Shevri (*Sesbania sesban L.*)

25. *Acacia tortilis*

Figures

2.1(a). C3 photosynthesis (PGA or 3 carbon compound as a
         primary product)

2.1(b)   C4 photosynthesis (Malate & Aspartate or 4 carbon compound

         as a primary product) Both types of photosynthesis path
         ways

2.1(c). CAM (Crassulacean Acid Metabolism) photosynthesis
         (4 carbon compound/organic acid produced in darkness)

9.1. Soil and plant succession/development, where grass is
      the final climax in well developed soil

10.1. Sequential degradation and improvement of Grassland
       types of the world

10.1. Climatic regions of Grasslands of India

10.2. Koeppen's world climate (Trewarth's1954-68)

10.3. Koeppen's world climates (Trewarth's 1954 and 1968)

10.4. The grass cover of tropical Africa.

10.5. Koeppen's world climates (Trewarth's 1954 and 1968)

10.6. Major grazing lands of the earth (Moore, 1966)

15.1. Yield response to supply of nutrient in soil

15. 2. Concentration of nutrient in plant and growth/yields.

15. 3. Schematic outline of nitrogen cycle

List of Tables

5.1. Important species and cultivars with distinct characters

5.2. Nutrient Requirement Based on Plant Analysis

11.1 Nutrients Loss in Hay Process (%)

11.2 Nutrient losses in process (%)

13.1 Continents and Area (%) Under Rangeland

13.2 Area Under Rangelands

15.3 Average Concentration of Mineral Nutrients in Plant Shoot Dry Matter (DM), Sufficient for Adquate Growth

15.4 Nutrients in Soils and their Fertility Range

17.1 Soil, Water and Nutrient Losses at 1% Slope at Kota Clay Soil

17.2 Run-off and Soil loss under Different Systems of Land Use in Ranchi (India)

17.3 Runoff and Soil loss on 9% Slop in Dehradoon during Monsoon and Dry

17.4 Soil Loss under Different Cropping Sequences in Hyderabad

17.5 Grass Specis for Different Regions of Rajasthan Under Different Rainfall

Chapter 1

Introduction

The foundation of a sustainable farming system rests on the pillars of the philosophy of 'holism'. The concept of holism is embodied in our scripture and tradition. Since, stability of the soil-forage/food crops-animal/human chain entails the very survival of the mankind on this planet which is evident from the *Sanskrit* text of 1500 B C.

"Upon This Handful Of Soil Our Survival depends

Husband It And It Will Grow Our Food, Our Fuel, our Shelter And

Surrounded With Bounty.

Abuse It And Soil Will Collapse and Die Taking Man With It"

The importance of forages and livestock in our agriculture system is also highlighted in an ancient Tamil proverb:

" No fodder No cattle

No cattle No manure

No Manure No crop"

Increasing trends in demand of food round the world to feed the swelling human population is taunting the Agricultural scientists to accept resolve the challenge. The situation in most of the developing Asian countries in general and in whole of the Africa in particular, is possing a threat to world peace under the present erratic nature of the climate and over exploitation of the natural resources in unscientific manner. The demographic compulsion encountered with unexpected drastic harass in productivity of soils due to harvesting of high input requiring high yielding genotypes in absence of inadequate soil care has put the soil in a very vunerable conditions.

The continuous increasing trends in imbalance application of chemical sources of nutrients without organic sources has virtually robbed the soil wealth to such an extent that the fertility and production potential of the soil have lost. The day is not very far off to result in a complete failure of the crop alike to that of bouncing of the cheque in absence of sufficient money in the Bank account, of cource the soil is also a Bank of the plant nutrients.

A marked reduction in liverslock wealth in general and draft animals in particular, speaks the future of sustainable faming system in India in absence of adequate availability of compost, has curtailed the farming system to a susceptible cropping system.

Though, the country has secured the first position in milk production however , it stands only at the 80th position to per capita availability of milk (245g) which is even below to the world average (267g). We are rearing half fed animals since the country is only meeting the 37% of green and 77% of dry fodder demands of the livestock as such only 4.0% of cultivable land is under forage production system to feed the 15% of the world livestock population or rather we are rearing cattle as a by-product fed on farm byproducts. Besides other factors, poor management condition is one of the factors responsible for duration and production potential of milk to per lactation of our cows. On an average, a cow in Israel, produces 9,000 lt. milk/cow/lactation while in India it is merely 900 lt./cow/lactation (10%) speaks the level of priority given to this industry.

Ignorance of forage-livestock system and giving top priority to cereals in general and rice production in particular in rice growing countries has led these countries below the poverty line. The world statistic of agricultural system very clearly revealed that except Japan, no any other rice growing countries stand among the 20 rich countries of the world. The countries which have given the least option to forage-livestock system, their majority of families stand below the poverty line. As such, China stands at the 103 and India at 117th position in GDP. Thus these countries need to put up at least 10% of their cultivable land under forage production for an economically and biologically viable farming system.

Therefore, a sustainable farming system for a viable healthy society, demands an adequate addition of organic sources of nutrients for stability in food crop production system, is the only way out to meet the present day challenges through proper management of animal wealth with sufficient production of nutritious forages. It will cater the need of the society by supplying adequate quantity and quality of food materials on one hand and sufficient quantity of milk and milk products to our people on the other. As such, a healthy soil produces healthy crops and healthy society.

Some of the important terms used in forage and grassland management system can be defined and deduced as under.

Forage

Forage is a vegetable or green food for feeding the domestic animals, which includes pasturage, browse, hay and silage.

Forage Crops

The crops, which are grown primarily for feeding the livestock to be either harvested for hay, silage or green feed or directly grazed by animals.

Fodder

Fodder is the above ground part of nearly mature corn or sorghum in the fresh or cured form. It includes byproducts of all the food crops *viz;* straw of cereals and pulses etc.

Thus, if a maize crop is cut in green stage after completion of vegetative phase or just before 50% flowering stage is termed as a forage maize/crop. If, the same maize crop is grown for grain or cobs production and stalk as a byproduct is fed to the livestock, is termed as a fodder. Hence, depending upon the objective, a food crop may also be known as a forage crop. Thus, if, a wheat or rice crop is cut before flowering and fed to the livestock, is also known as a forage crops since, it is entirely dependent on the primary objective.

Therefore, a forage crop is more nutritious as compared to a fodder since in later, the nutritive value in majority is transferred to the grains.

Forage Acre

A hypothetical acre with a 10/10 density of forage that can be utilized to the limits of the physiological endurance of the vegetation is termed as forage acre.

Forage Acre = Forage Acre Factor x Surface Area

Forage Acre Factor (PAF)

is an expression of relative forage value which is a product of average density (by type and sub-type) of range forage x Proper-Use-Factor (average weight palatability).

or, PAF = Density (%) x PUF.

Forage Value

The rank of a range plant for grazing animals under proper management, expresses in proper-Use-Factor. or, PUF < 1.

Proper-Use-Factor/Palatability Factor

The percentage weight (some times height) at which the available plant species are grazed when the range is used properly.

Grazing/Carrying Capacity: The number of animal units that can be maintained on a unit area for a stated period of time without over grazing is known as grazing/carrying capacity.

Or, Carrying capacity = Area/ Animal Unit.

Reconnaissance

It is a type of grazing survey done in a special sense.

Grassland

It is very definitely one of a number of "**seral**" phases of vegetation.

"**Seral**" is an ecological development as an orderly series of events in which one association acts as a nursery to its immediate successor. The whole series of seasonal phases from first to last, is referred to as the 'sere' and grassland forms, one of the characteristic phase in that 'sere'

Since, in grasslands, grass is the dominant partner in comparision to legumes hence it is designated as grassland. Migration of grasses from one place to another is easier than legumes due to small and light seed weight. Among other characters, it is one of the favourable characters which enable it to dominate in association with legumes.

Grassland Geography

Since geography is the study of the natural features of the earth's surface, including topography, climate, soil and vegetation hence grassland geography is very definitely is the science that describes the surface of the earth and its associated biological characteristics, here refers to grasses. Therefore, distribution of grasslands is the result of climate, edaphic, topography, fire and biotic interference.

Biome

Biome is a biotic community of geographysical extent characterized by distinctiveness in the life forms of the important climax species. It is based on the life form of the most important plants (trees, grasses and shrubs).

Some other defined biomes, as units of study of interaction between different communities of the area and hence biome ecology is the out come of the interaction among community 1 (climax) dominant species say, A, community 2 approaching to climate and community 3 under early succession.

A biome is the complex of communities maintained by the climate of the region and characterized by a distinctive type of vegetation. Therefore, biome is a bigger unit than community, constitutes the great regions of the world distinguished by on ecological basis as: Tundras biomes, forest biomes, grassland biomes and scrubs or desert biomes.

As per succession theory it is one of the stages of homeostasis of organisms:

Population → communities → ecosystems → landscapes → biome → ecosphere or the stage that comes just before ecosphere.while homeostasis is the sequence of events occurring one after another:

Organ systems → organs → tissues → cells → molecules → atoms. Both sequences occur in either direction.

Classification of Forage Crops

The forage crops are broadly classified as tropical and temperate forages which are further classified as grasses and legumes as well as annual and perennial on the basis of their growth habit.

Climatic Classification of Forage Crops: The forage crops of the world are broadly classified in two groups as:

a. Tropical forages b. Temperate forages

(a) Tropical forages

The forage crops which are grown under the tropical conditions are grown during monsoon period in India is known as *Kharif* forage crops. The same crop species are also cultivated in summer season under irrigated conditions. These may be annuals or perennials grasses and legumes.

Grasses/ Cereals

Annuals

Deenanath grass (*Pennisetum pedicellatum*)
Jowar (*Pennisetum typhoid*)
Bajra (*Sorghum bicolor*)
Sudan grass (*Sorghum sudanensis*)
Maize (*Zea mays*)
Teosinte (*Euchalena mexicana*)

Perennials

Napier/ Elephant grass (*Pennisetum purpureum*)
Thin Napier/Mission grass *(Pennisetum polystchyon)*
Gamba/Sadabahar grass (*Andropogon gayanus*)
Para grass (*Brachiaria mutica*)
Palasid grass (*B. brizantha*)
Signal grass (*B. decumbens*)
Guines grass (*Panicum maximum*)
Nandi/ Cojungula grass (*Setaria sphacelata decumbens*)
Anjan/Buffel grass (*Cenchrus ciliaris*)
Bermuda/ Doob grass (*Cynodan dactylon)*
Spear grass (*Heterpogon contortus)*

Legumes

Annuals

Cowpea (*Vigna unguiculata*)
Rice bean (*Vigna umbellate*)
Moth bean (*Phaseolus aconitifolius*)
Lablab bean (*Lablab purpureus*)
 Townsville stylo (*Stylosanthes humilis*)

Cassia (*Cassia rotendifollia*)
Pigeon pea/Arhar *(Cajanus cajan)*
Kudaliya (*Desmodium spp.*)

Perennials

Brazilian Lucerne (*Stylosanthes guianensis*)
River Hunter Lucerne/Caribbean stylo (*S. hamata*)
Shrubby stylo (*S. scabra*)
Siratro (*Macroptillium atropurpureum*)
Centro (*Centrosema pubescens*)
Puerarea (*Pueraria phaseoloides)*
Calpo (*Calpogonium muconoides*)
Glycine (*Glycine wightti*)
Kudzu vine (*Pureraria labata)*)
Peanut (*Arachis glabrata*)

b. Temperate Forages

Forage crops which are cultivated in temperate regions of the world or under low temperature conditions is termed as temperate forage crops. These crops are grown in India as a winter crops and commonly known as *Rabi* forage crops. Such crops are also cultivated at high altitudes in the tropical to sub-tropical countries, termed as highlands forages mostly as annuals.

Grasses/ cereals

Annuals

Oats (*Avena sativa*)
Kikuyu grass (*Pennisetum cladestinum*)
Ryegrass (*Lolium multiflorum*)
Barley (*Hordeum vulgare*)

Perennials

Perennial Rye grass (*Lolinum perenne*)
Kentucky Blue grass (*Poa pratensis*)
Rescue grass (*Bromus canthorticus*)
Orchard grass (*Dactylis glomerata*)
Reed Canary grass (*Phalaris arudinacea)*
Harding grass (*Phalaris aquatica*)

Tall Fescue (*Festuca arundinacea*)

Timody (*Phelum pretense*)

Legumes

Annuals

Egyptian clover (*Trifolium alexandrinum*)

Alsike clover (*T. hybridum*)

White/Ladino clover (*T. repens*)

Red clover (*T. pretense*)

Crimson clover (*T. incarnatum*)

Subterranium clover (*T. subterraneum*)

Shaftal (*T. resupinatum*)

Strawberry clover (*T. fragiferum*)

Lucerne/Alfalfa (*Medicago sativa*)

Vetches (*Vicia spp.*)

Perennials: shrubs/trees;

Subabool (*Leucaena leucocephala*)

Hedge Lucerne (*Desmenthus vurgatus*)

Agathi (*Sesbania grandiflora*)

Gliricidia (*Gliricidia sepium*)

Shevri (*Sesbania sesban*)

Callindra (*Calliandra calothyrsus*)

Acasia (*Acasia tortilis*)

Miscellaneous Forages (*Non-grass / non-legume*)

Amaranthus (*Amaranthus spp.*)

Chinese cabbage (*Brassica chinensis*)

Forage beet (*Beta vulgaris* var. sativa)

Forage carrot (*Daucus carota* var. sativa)

Rape/mustard/choumollier(*Brassica spp.*)

Turnips (*Brassica ropa*)

Sweet potato (*Ipomoea batatas*)

Chapter 2

Grasses and Legumes

In general, forage species are more competant in utilization of natural resources as compared to food crops. Among forage crops, grasses being a C4 species, can exploit the soil and climate conditions more efficiently. Grasses due to their well developed fine root system can extract the soil moisture and plant nutrients more effectively than legumes due to low thresh hold value for the different nutrients as well as due to their total CEC however, CEC of forage legumes to per unit root surface area is 2-4 times higher than grasses but total CEC is less to grasses because of limited root system.

Grasses can also utilize the increases in CO_2 concentration and atmospheric temperature to increase their productivity where as legumes may suffer such conditions. Therefore, in total, forages are more sustainable under stress conditions than food crops. Some of the differences between grasses and legumes are summerised under the following different headings.

Grasses	Legumes
Family: Gramineae (Poaceae)or Grass family has 450 genera and Over 6,000 species **A. Morphological:** Habit: Annual or perennial herbs, rarely shrubs or trees usually of a hollow cylindrical culms.	**Family:** Leguminosae has 3 sub-familes of which forage legumes belong to sub-family, Papilionoideae **Habit:** Herbs, shrubs or trees often climbers **Roots:** Tap root systems with nodules possessing nitrogen fixing bacteria *contd...*

Contd...

Grasses	Legumes
Roots: Adventitious root system, some may have rhizomes (Johson grass), rooting at every nodes (Bermuda grass) and underground runners (*Panicum spps.*)	**Roots:** Tap root systems with nodules possessing nitrogen fixing bacteria
Stems: Hollow cylindrical stems but solid in food crops; maize, sorghum and pearlmillet. Very hard and tall woody in bamboo with absence of branching.	**Stems:** Hollow to solid stems with branching, erect to prostrate, runners to climbers having stem and leaves tendrils, some with hooks and even twinings (*Dolichos*).
Leaves: Leaves are arranged alternately at the nodes and internodes are covered with leaf sheaths, auricle may be fully developed (barley) or rudimentary (wheat) or even absent (oat). Leaf blades are erectophyll with parallel veination, entire margin and may be covered with hairs. In some species leaf margin may be enough panic (*Panicum* and *Saccharum* spps.)	**Leaves:** The planophyll leaves are arranged on the branches as unipinnate (peripinnate and imparipinnate), bipinnate or tripinnate or decompound may be pedicelleted or sessile with reticulate veination and serrate, dentate or entire margins In some species leaf blades may be covered with hairs and gummy materials to reduce transpiration and for the same some species perform xeric movement.
Inflorescence: It is spike or spike of spikelet, one sessile and pedicelleted or even subdivided into branches is known as panicle. Bisexual or unisexual flowers grouped into one to a dozen of small florets, glumes bear awn, each floret has two bracts as lemma (outer) and palea (inner) within which two to three lodicules are situated. Vegetative and reproductive phases are distinct, and even flowering and fruiting are synchronized leading to higher yield compared to legumes.	**Inflorescence:** Flowers either on the top or on the axil with combination of petals as one standard, two wing and two kells. Calyx: Sepals 4 or 5 free or united Corolla: Petals 4 or 5, one standard, two wings and one kell. **Androecium:** 10 stamens or several. **Gynoecium:** Carpel 1 with superior ovary. Flowering, fruiting and even vegetative growth are simultaneous which results to low productivity due to translocation of energy in both directions i.e., vegetative and reproductive phases.
Androecium : Stamens 3 or 6 with versatile anthers	
Gynoecium: Carpel 1, ovary superior, unilocular with single ovule and 2 stigmas.	
Fruits: Caryopsis, monocot of which sheath does not come out during germination and embryo situated outside of the endosperm having hypogeal germination.	**Fruit:** Very well identified with pods. Each pod may have one to several dicot fleshy seeds from oval to kidney shaped which has epigeal germination.

Contd...

Grasses	Legumes
B. Physiological:	
Since, cambium tissues are absent hence secondary growth does not occur. Presence of kranz cells and chloroplast act in re-trapping of CO_2 during photosynthesis (Hatch and Slack, 1966).Since, the primary product of photosynthesis in grasses contains 4 carbon compounds such as malate and aspirate hence, such species are known as C_4 plants.	Presence of cambium tissue facilitates secondary growth while absence of kranz anatomy and chloroplasts does not help to re-trap CO_2 during photosynthesis. Since, the primary product of photosynthesis in legumes and non-grasses are 3 carbon compound i.e., PGA (3-Phosphoglyceric acid) hence, such species are known as C_3-plants.

The C-3 Cycle

This cycle (Fig. 2.1a) envolves 4 reactions: Carboxylation of RuBP to 2PGA, phosphorylation of PGa to1,3-DPGA, reduction of 1,3-DPGA toG3P and finaly the regeneration of RuBP from G3P in which chemical energy is derived from ATP. The net reaction can be as,

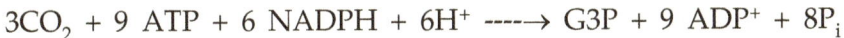

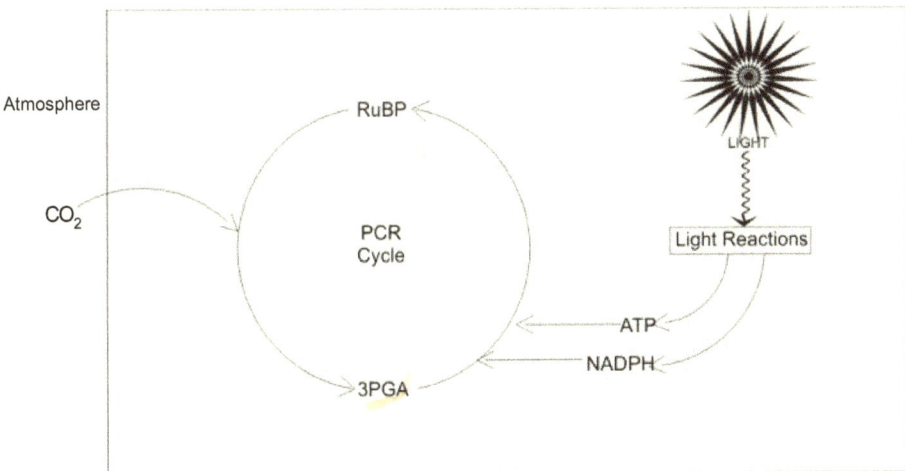

$$3CO_2 + 9\ ATP + 6\ NADPH + 6H^+ \longrightarrow G3P + 9\ ADP^+ + 8P_i$$

Fig. 2.1(a): C3 photosynthesis (PGA or 3 carbon complound as a primary product)

The C 4- Cycle

The differences in C4 plant (Fig.2.1b) is the original carboxylation of CO_2. The CO_2 acceptor is the 3-carbon compound phosphoenol pyruvate (PEP) and the product is the 4-carbon compound oxaloacetate (OAA) which occurs in mesophyll cells and the bundle sheath..

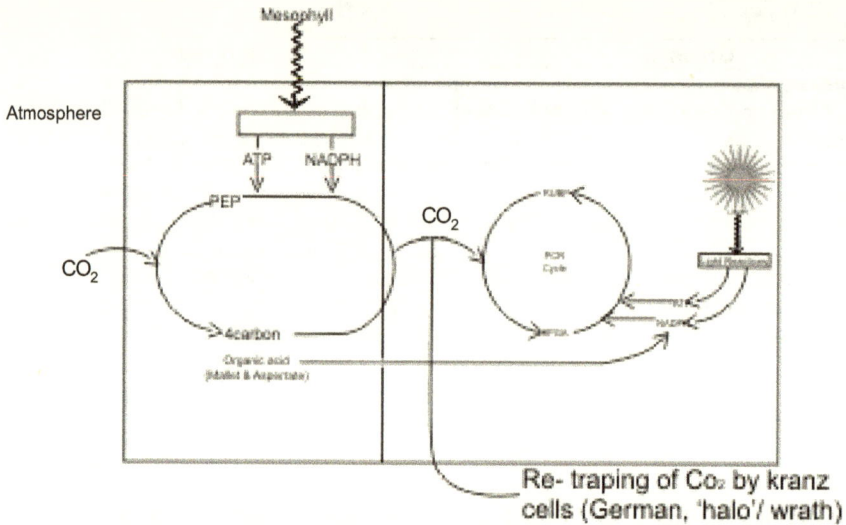

Fig. 2.1(b): C4 photosynthesis (Malate & Aspartate or 4 compound as a primary product) Both types of photosynthesis path ways

Crassulacean acid metabolism (CAM)

In such plants (Fig. 2.1c) the stomata are open in the night and the level of malic acid in the vacole increases while in the day the stomata closes and the level of malic acid falls. CO_2 uptake predominatly occurs in the dark. CAM plants contain the enzymes of C4 plants and carboxylation of PEP to malate in the dark when the stomata are open and a pool of malate is formed.

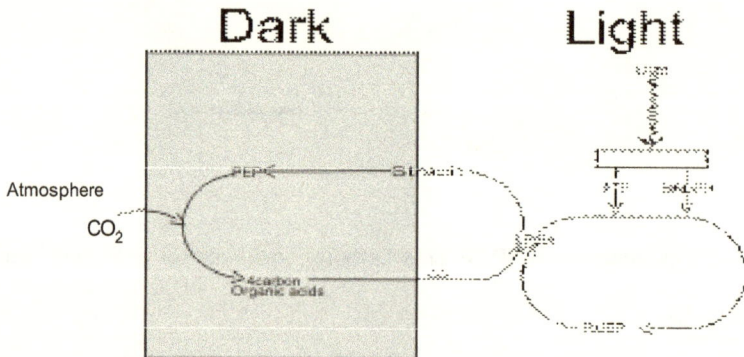

Fig. 2.1(c): CAM (Crassulacean Acid Metabolism) photosynthesis (4 carbon compound/organic acid produced in darkness)

On the basis of primary product during photosynthesis as discussed above in brief (Fig.a, b and c), the plants are broadly classified into three categories. As such, if the primary stable product of photosynthesis of a plant, contains 3- carbon compound ie, Pyruvate Glyceric Acid (PGA), the plant is known as C_3 plant. The example of this group includes main food crops viz; rice, wheat and legumes. Accordingly, if the primary stable product of photosynthesis of a plant contains 4-carbon compounds ie, Aspartate by Guinea grass and millets while Mallet by Maize, Sorghum and Sugarcane the plants are known as C_4 plants. All the tropical grasses including bamboos and major food crops like maize, sorghum and sugarcane belong to this group. The third type of plants belong to family Crassulaceae and hence photosynthetic process is known as Crassulacean Acid Metabolism (CAM) in which the acidification continue to occur during day as well as during night and stomata opens only during night results in less loss of water. Pineapples and aspergilus as well as arid plant like cacti are the some plants belong to this type. It requires average maximum day and night temperatures of 35°C and 15°C, respectively for maximum net assimilation but xeric species may survive even above 50°C. Some of the plant species have both C_3 and C_4 path ways of photosynthesis. Though, the barley and pea are the C_3 plants however, green pigment of barley panicle and pods of peas perform C_4 cycle. Since, majority of forage grasses belong to C_4 and legumes as C_3 hence, their responses to change in atmospheric conditions (CO_2, temperature and solar radiation) are given in brief.

B1. Photosynthetic responses to CO_2 concentration on legumes (C_3) and grasses (C_4)

a.	Grasses may show growth stimulation through greater water use efficiency and leaf area as compared to legumes.	a.	Low water efficiency of legumes does not show growth stimulation as grasses.
b.	High sink capacity of C_4 plants has the highest response to CO_2 enrichment with 30-40 % more biomass production as compared to C_3 species.	b.	It does not happen in C_3 species due to low sink capacity.
c.	Grasses use to continue acidification at CO_2 concentration as low as 5 ppm and as high as 500ppm.	c.	Legumes usually ceased to photosynthesis process if, CO_2 concentration falls below 20ppm and above 350 ppm.
d.	C_4 exhibits photosynthesis from 19 m mol /m^2/s to 65 m mol/m^2/s of CO_2.	d.	C_3 exhibits photosynthesis rate $1/3^{rd}$ i.e., from 6m mol/m^2/s to 22m mol/m^2/s of CO_2.
e.	Transpiration ratio of 200:350 indicates less loss in net energy	e.	Transpiration ratio 500:1000 indicates high loss in net energy

B2. Photosynthetic responses to temperature on C$_3$ and C$_4$ plants:

a. Grasses normally operate at saturating concentration of CO_2 as a result, Rubisco (Ribulose 1, 5 biphosphate carbooxylate – oxygenase) is more sensitive to temperature as compared to C$_3$ Photo synthesis and continues at 30-45^{0}C	a. Most of the legumes, the assimilation is decreased when temperature falls below 15^{0}C normal temperature is from 20-25^{0}C as such Rubisco is less sensitive to temperature
b. A marked rise in photo synthesis with increasing temperature under high light intensity occurs in grasses.	b. In legumes the assimilation rate is increased at higher CO_2 concentration only upto 30^{0}C.
c. Though, most of the grasses are absent from temperate environment however, it can survive at low temperature for some time.	c. C$_3$ plants, at high temperature coincided with low light intensity is injurious to plant due to higher rate of photo respiration.
d. At temperature less than 12^{0}C grasses (C4) are prone to chilling injury but photo synthesis is continued even temperature upto 40^{0}C.	d. High light intensity increases photo synthesis upto 30^{0}C and thereafter it is drastically reduced.
e. If performs better acidification above 30^{0}C, even it is continued at 50^{0}C in sorghum.	e. CO_2 fixation is declined above 30^{0}C even though other conditions are normal and thus several plant species die above 40^{0}C and some at 45^{0}C.
f. At 0 – 5^{0}C, C4 plants develop Chlorotic strips **(Faris banding)** across the leaf blades	f. Such extreme condition of temperature is fatal for C$_3$ plants.
g. Some *Cacti spps* (CAM plants) even survive at 50^{0}C and can sustain for one hour at 70^{0}C.	

B3. Light intensity in relation to C$_3$ and C$_4$ plants;

When light is emitted, it behaves as through its energy which is divided into discrete units or particles called **quantum**. The energy carried by a proton is represented by Eq.

$$Eq = hc/ \; / = hv: Eq = 4.56 \times 10^{-19} \text{ J proton}$$

Quantum Yield: It is the photosynthetic efficiency measured as quantum yield of oxygen evolution, is the inverse of the quantum requirement, that is, number of molecules of oxygen evolved to per proton absorbed.

$$Q10 = \frac{RT + 10}{RT}$$

The temperature response to chemical and biological reactions is characterized by comparing the rate of reaction at the two temperatures 10°C apart, a value known as Q10.

The value of Q10 for enzyme-catalyzed reactions is about 2, that the rate of reaction will be double for each 10°C rise in temperature.

In general, optimum wave- length for photosynthesis for all the plants happens to be between 400-700 *nm* (1 *nm* = 10^{-9} m) while 555 *nm* is the optimum, wave length for the maximum visibility for a normal man. Tropical C_4 plant has the maximum photosynthesis at 400 *nm* and continue photosynthesis without saturation as the average energy received at this wave length is more than 290 kJmole/proton while temperate C_3 plant at or nearer to 700 *nm* and shows saturation below 500 micro-mole of proton as the average energy received at this wave length is less than 85 kJmole/ proton. Therefore, high intensity radiant energy is good for tropical grasses whereas low radiant energy is ideal for temperate legumes. Photosynthesis rate or CO2 fixation rate to per unit leaf area of C_4 plants in general and to that of sorghum is the highest.

Bio-mass and Seed Production Potential of Grass and Legume

The green herbage production of grasses in general is higher than legumes except to that of multi-cut legumes. The dry matter content in grasses is higher but legumes are more in protein content and several other nutrients. In general, forages are shy in seed production. The seed production potential of several perennial grasses is very low as compared to legumes, but seed production in cereal forages is higher than both grain as well as forage legumes.

Chapter 3

Tropical Forage Cereals

Sorghum/Jowar (*Sorghum bicolor*)

Jowar(*Sorghum bicolor* (L.) Moech, of family *Poaceae* is a tall annual or perennial native to Asia and Africa with long, flat semi-erectophyl leaves. Five jointed cluster of recemes are the parts of inflorescence, spikelets in pairs with one fully developed sterile and pedicellated, but the other one is sessile and fertile. Flowers consisted of 2 large lodicules, 3 stamens, 2 styles. In cultivated types, the grain size is of obovate but in wild types it is linear-oblong. The colours of the grains vary from red, brown, yellow or even white.

History and Distribution

The name sorghum is originated from an Italian word '*Sorgo*' means 'rising above' specifying its tall erect growth character is also known as great millet. It is grown through out the world and in India it is known as *Jowar* and in Africa as Black-Amber. It is acknowledged with the Great Millet due to the fact that it is the most important cereals among millets. Since, water requirement of sorghum is less hence, it is the dominant crop in arid and semi-arid regions of the world. It is intensively grown in USA, Australia, Africa and Manchuria. In India, it is the main cereal in Deccan plateau and as well as the main forage crop as it shares 50 percent of total forage area and production of the country comprising of Madhya Pradesh, Andhra Pradesh, Chhatisgarh, Maharastra, Tamil Nadu and Karnataka. It is also grown in UP, Bihar,

Rajsthan, Punjab and Haryana to some extent as a forage and grain crop. In UP and Bihar it is the main forage crop during the early monsoon as it is sown either in summer or with pre-monsoon rain.

Climate and Soils

Among the cultivated crops, sorghum as a C4 plant is the most efficient species to harvest the solar radiation and assimilation continued at low to high CO_2 concentrations and at temperature 40°C but can sustain even at 50°C. Temperature below 15°C and elevations above 1500 m from sea level are not conducive for normal growth. It is mainly a crop suitable for rain-fed and dry-land agro-eco-systems. As it favours arid to semiarid regions of the tropics, sub-tropics and extended to sub-temperate conditions. Soils with heavy texture of both black and red with high water retaining capacity are favourable. Though, it is a drought resistant plant but it can tolerate water logging to some extent. It is also tolerant to medium acidity, alkalinity and salinity.

Package of Practices

Though, ploughing of black Alfisols does not influence the productivity but ploughing after summer rain, controls the weeds and facilitates better germination and crop growth. Under drylands situations, one ploughing with soil turning plough followed by 2 with blade harrows or cultivators may be sufficient to make a medium tilth.

Nutrients Requirements

Crop grown in low rainfall area is hardly fertilized but high rainfall areas with low soil moisture retaining capacity where, dryland practices are followed, 5-7 tonnes/ha of FYM along with 20-25 kg P_2O_5/ha as basal followed by 20-25 kg N/ha is top-dressed at 6 weeks crop or preferably just after rain at that time. If, it is at all cultivated under irrigated conditions or areas of sufficient rainfall with soil having good moisture holding capacity but devoid of water logging can be well manured with 10 tonnes/ha of FYM + 25 kg N/ha + 20kg P_2O_5/ha as basal followed by 30kg N/ha 4-5 weeks crop age.

Varieties and Sowing

Since the establishment of Indian Grassland and Fodder Research Institute (IGFRI) at Jhansi and starting of All India Coordinated Project on Forage Crops, a large number of varieties of different forage have been released. In these varieties the concentration of HCN is low as compared to old one, even though it is advised to cut and feed the livestock at 50% flowering stage and other multicut varieties first cut at 55 days after emergence.and subsequent cuts at 40 days. Crop sown in summer season may contain more HCN. Therefore, the first cut should be taken preferably after rain which washes the highly soluble HCN, in absence of rain the cut chaps should be washed after keeping in water for over night.

A lage number of single (over 20), double (5) and multicut (15) varieties with variable characteristics have been evolved on national and state levels.

Single cut varieties

Variety	Character and Yield
Pusa Chari-1	Resistant to lodging, drought and pests, very responsive to nutrients with 30 t/ha green and 9t/ha dry matter yields
Pusa Chari-6	Performed well in all the sorghum growing area of the country with 32-34 t GF/ha and 11-13 t DM/ha
Pusa Chari-23	A very high yielder for growing in entire sorghum growing regions with 40-45 t GF/ha and 15-16 t DM/ha
Pusa ChariHybrid-106 (HC-106)	Tall type (235 cm), high tillering, leafy with green mid rib. Green leaves with semi planofix long (75-78 cm) and broad (5-6 cm). Partially sterile flower but resistant to diseases as well as of stem borer and fly shoot. Cut at 50-60 days of age for forage (6.5-7.0 t GF/ha and about 2 t DM/ha). Seeding to seed formation in about 100 days,
MP Chari	Suitable for Central, Eastern and North India Mature in 110 days and gives 30 t GF/ha and 10 t DM/ha
Jawahar Chari-6	Suitable for medium to heavy soils of central India. Pearly white bold seed. Tall plant (> 300 cm), resistant to diseases More than 70 t GF/ha amd 20 t DM/ha
SL- 44	Hybrid from JS-263 x SSG59-3 and suitable for NW region.
HC-136	Ideal for irrigated conditions. Tall with broad leaves matures in 140 days, resistant to leaf diseases, low HCN and tannine contents. It is juicy with high protein and digestibility. About 40 t GF/ha and 10-11 j DM/ha
Haryanana Chari-171	A cross of SPV-8X x IS-4776. Good for irrigated conditions in monsoon and summer seasons. Tall plant with long and broad leaves resistant to diseases with 32-35 t GF/ha and 9-10 t DM/ha.
Haryana Chari-260	Tall , juicy but not sweet, good for hay, early maturing with about 30 tGF/ha and 10 t DM/ha

Contd...

Variety	Character and Yield
HC-308	Tall plant, sweet stem, long-broad leaves, resistant to diseases with high yield up to 44 t GF/ha and 14 t DM/ha
Haryana Jowar-513	Product of S-305(PJ x SPV-80) x HC-136, is 250-260 cm tall, mid-rib white, long semi-compact panicle, resistant to gray leaf spot, zonet leaf spot and shooty stripe. More than 45 t GF/ha and 12 t DM/ha
UP Chari-1 (IS4776)	Developed from a single plant selection from *Durra caudatum*, for dry area with low HCN can be fed at any growth stage, medium yield (33t GF and 8 t DM/ha.
UP Chari-2	A cross of Vidisha-60-1 x IS 6953 followed by pedigree selection. For late sown conditions in low rainfall areas with about 38 tGF/ha
Pant Chari-4	350 cm tall, purple pigment with dark green leaves (62 cm) with light green mid-rib. 45-48 tGF/ha and 12-13 tDM/ha. Good for kharif season
Rajasthan Chari-1	A cross of CSVG x NCL3, resistant to stem borer, non-lodging with 45 t GF/ha and 12 t DM/ha
Rajasthan Chari-2 (SU-45)	Selected from local sorghum, resistant to stem borer with high digestibility. 30 t GF/ha and 8 t DM/ha
Gujarat Fodder Sorghum-5	Early maturing for arid and semi-arid areas in kharif. 275 cm tall thin stem. Ear head loose, pearly white grain. Resistant to diseases and grain mold with 38 t GF/ha and 14 t DM/ha
MFSH-3	A cross of 531 Yx SG 101, suitable for Maharastra with very high yield of 65 t GF/ha and 14 t DM/ha
Proagro Chari (SSG-988)	Product of private company, ideal for whole India

Double cut varieties

CO-27	This is a drought resistant variety of loose panicle with blackish purple glumes enclosing seed. It becomes ready for first cut at two months and next after 40-45 days in southern states and gives 40 t GF/ha with about 10% protein.
Gujarat Forage Sorghum Hybrid-1 (GFSH-1)	Developed through hybridization (3600A x IS-4776) is 240-260 cm tall, 11.5 cm thick stem 75-80 cm X 4.7-7.2 cm leaf size of white seeded. It is succulent and moderately salt tolerant gives 65 t GF/ha in 2 cuts, grown in Gujrat and southern states.

Multi cut varieties

SSG 59-3 (Meethi Sudan)	It is derived from pedigree selection of non-sweet sudan grass x IS-263, is a tall profused fast growing type. It is suitable for both drought and water logged conditions. Sweet and succulent with 75 t GF/ha and 22 t DM/ha is cultivated in north zone.
Jawahar Chari-69	Developed from hybridization (K-38 x J-98) followed by pedigree method of selection is 250 cm tall, long-narrow leaf and seed covered with black glumes. First cut at 55-60 days and subsequent cut at an interval of 40-45 days. In 4-5 cuts under irrigated conditions and 2 cuts as rainfed produces 55 t GF/ha and 15 t DM/ha in M.P.
PCH-106 Hybrid	A profused tillering fast regenerating capacity gives 65 t GF/ha in 3-4 cuts in north region.
Punjab Sudex Chari-1	A product of intervarital hybridization (2077 A x SGI-87) is grown in Punjab
Pant Chari-5 (UPFS-32)	The plants are 245 cm tall, semi-crect, tan type, highly juicy and internodes are fully enclosed. The leaves are 74 cm long and 6.2 cm broad with light green mid rib. The panicles are cylindrical, semi-compact, glumes are straw coloured. The seeds are pearly white, medium bold, soft and round. It is highly resistant to anthracnose zonate leaf spot and other foliar diseases. The nutritional qualities are good with protein content (6.6%), digestibility (47.7% and low HCN (100 ppm). Average yield of green fodder 48. t/ha, dry fodder 13.4 t/ha and seed18 q/ha.
CHS-20MF (UPMCH-1101)	This variety is developed by interspecific hybridization (2219AxUPMC 503) for cultivation in medium irrigated summer and rainfed conditions of Uttar Pradesh, Uttrakhand. Haryana. Rajasthan, Punjab, Bihar and Gujarat. It has low HCN content and is highly resistant to foliar diseases and lodging under natural conditions. It is tolerant to drought and water logging. It is tall (215cm), tan and has medium thick juicy stem with many basal tillers and long and medium broad semi-/crect stay-green leaves. This hybrid shows fast regeneration after cutting.
Pant Chari-6 (UPMCH-503)	This variety was developed from selection in Zimbabwe generplasm line FC-438401. The variety has been recommended for cultivation in Uttrakhand state under rainfed conditions during kharif season and under irrigated conditions in summer season. It reaches mid bloom in 65-70 days and matures in 105-110 days. The plants are tall, erect, tan pigmented and stem is sweet and juicy (TSS>7%).The seed is red, semi-bold and circular in shape. It provides 80-100 t/ha green forage and 25-35t/ha dry matter and 18-20 q/ha seed yield.

Contd...

Pant Chari Hybrid-109 (PCH-109)	It is a multi cut hybrid developed for cultivation during early summer and normal Kharif under timely sown rainfed areas in Delhi.The plants are 225 cm tall.semi crect, stay green type, leafy (13/plant) with juricy stem. Its leaves are 83cm long and 6.5 cm broad with dull green mid rib. The panicles are semi- loose, the grains are creamy white. It attains 50% flowering in 60 days and matures in 101 days. The variety is tolerant to major foliar diseases, shoot fly and stem borer. It produces 82 t/ha green forage and 21 t/ha dry forager.
Pusa Chari-615	This variety is a derivative of the cross between Pusa chari 40xPusa chari 67. It has been recommended for cultivation during early summer and kharif seasons of NCR Delhi. The variety mid blooms in 70 days and matures in 110 days. The plants are 300-320 cm tall and green type with 3-6 tillers in a plant. The leaves are dark green 75-85cm long and 5.0-6.5 cm wide. The leaf stem ratio is 0.35-0.45. The panicles are semi loose. It produces 70 t/ha green forage, 19.5 t/ha dry forage and 12q/ha seed. The protein content in forage is 8.1%, IVDMD 55.3% and HCN content 152 ppm. The variety is resistant to major foliar diseases and insect- pests.
Haryana Jowar-513 (S-513)	Thy variety is a derivative of S-305 (PJ-7R X SPV-80) X HC-136. It is recommended for cultivation in Haryana under timely sown/ normal fertility, irrigated conditions. The variety is ready for green fodder harvest in 100-110 day. The plants are 245 – 260 cm tall with white midrib leaves. The ear heads are very long, symmetrical and semi – compact. It is tolerant to major foliar diseases like gray spot (*Cercospora south*) and zonate leaf spot. The green forage yield of the variety is 49 t/ha and dry matter yield is 12 t/ha.
COFS-29	The variety was released in 2001 and developed by interspecific hybridization followed by pedigree method of selection (TNS 30 X S. sudhnese). It gives 5-6 cuts in one year at 60 days intervals. The leaves and stems are highly succulent in nature. It contains high protein (8.41%) and less crude fibre (34.0%). It attains 50% flowering in 65-70% days and ready for seed harvest in 105-110 days. The variety is recommended for cultivation in Tamil Nadu under irrigated conditions. The plants are 220 -250 cm tall with 2.5-3.0 cm stem girth, having 10-15 tillers/ plant. 80-105 leaves/plant of 75-90 x 3.5-4.6 cm size It is tolerant to shoot fly stem borer. Average yield of green fodder is 170 t/ha, 34.5 t/ha dry matter and seed yield is 5 q/ha.
Proagro Chari (SSG_988)	This is a hybrid (PFFI x PFG 2) x PFM 1..The variety is suitable for cultivation in Andhra Pradesh and N-W states of India. It is high tillering, thin stem, leafy dark green in colour producing 40-50 t/ha green fodder and 10 t/ha dry matter.

Contd...

| Hara Sona 855 | The variety has been notified for cultivation in sorghum growing areas in N-W India, is derived from the cross between (PFS5A x PFS5C) x PFS5R followed by pedigree method of selection. It is high tillering, thin stemmed, tall, multi- cut, high in protein content and low in HCN. The green fodder yield is 60-65t/ha. It is widely grown SSG hybrid in India. |
| Safed Moti (FSH-92079) | The variety was developed through hybridization (PSA93016 x FSR 93025) is recommended for cultivation in north India. High protein and low in HCN, gives 65-70 t/ha green fodder. |

Different countries and even different agro-climatic conditions of the same country, usually cultivate their own suitable genotypes.In East African countries, Sumac and white African varieties are the most popular. In Northern India, summer sown Jowar and feeding as forage in early monsoon season allow to grow rice as succeeding crop. In Deccan plateau region, it is grown as a main crop from July to November-December or even till February as a grain crop. In African low land it is cultivated from June to November.

Line dibbling of 15-20 kg seeds/ha behind the plough at 40 cm and 5 cm soil depth is followed for grain production but for forage purposes it is usually sown as broadcast with 60-70 kg seeds/ha or even higher amount, followed by one harrowing and planking.

Inter-culturing, Pests and Diseases Control

If, sorghum is grown as a food crop, maintaining right plant population with thinning is a must, especially under irrigated conditions but it is seldom done if, it is grown as a forage crop or grain crop under rain-fed and dryland conditions. However, for grain crop under irrigated conditions, first hoeing at one month and next just at flag leaf initiation stage with earthing- up gives a good yield.

Among the insects, stem borer at young stage and earhead bug at flowering period are the most common. It is better to uproot the affected plants of borers and burn them. Bugs can be effectively controlled by dusting with 1 percent Aldrin dust at milky stage.

Seed born disease like grain smut (*Sphacelotheca sorghii*), particularly the crop grown in cold season is very common.

In place of grains, a short grey sacs filled up with black powdery mass of fungal spores are found. This seed borne disease can be controlled by treating the seeds with Thirum, Agrosan GN, or any other present day fungicide @ 2g/kg of seeds.

Loose smut (*S. cruenta*) and head smut (*Sorosporium reilianum*) diseases are also common. Loose smut reduces the forage quality and further resulted in very low grain yields. Seed treatment with the fungicides, control the disease very effectively. Head smut is a soil borne disease; it changes the inflorescence into a large-whitish gall known as 'sorus'. Uprooting and burning of the affected plants before the scattering of the spores are advised.

Some of the bacterial diseases are often common. Among them, Downy mildew (*Scleropora sorghi*) in which, young leaves changes to yellow and then brown followed by appearance of white fungus on dorsal side of the leaves results in absence of earheads. Such soil borne disease can be only controlled by burning of the diseased plants.

In some parts of Asia and Africa, phanerogamic parasite (*Striga hermontheca* and *S. lutea*) are some times very common. The small seeds of this parasite remains in the soils and germinate along the crop seeds which latter develops haustoria and penetrates the crop roots. Thus, the plants show a scorched appearance and finally reduced yields. Application of 2, 4-D herbicide before seeding is very effective. Some disease resistant genotypes can be a better option to get away from this parasite.

Prussic Acid (HCN) Poisoning

Some of the varieties in general and old one in particular at early growth stage of plants develop prussic acid or HCN poisoning, is also known as Dhurian poisoning. It develops under high temperature conditions of hot summer months followed by moisture stress in some of the varieties at early stage of growth or at 5-7 leaves stage which is further removed by rain. Re-growth from a ratoon crop of sorghum, Sudan grass and Johson is more toxic than crops raised from seeds. For feeding such crop, the forage may be chaffed and put in water for over night. This will remove the loosely attached acid and let the forage free from toxic material.

Cutting Management

Single-cut early or late types can be cut at 50% flowering stage for green feeding while, milking stage will be ideal for silage purposes. In late multi-cut types, first cut can be taken just before the initiation of flag leaf and subsequent cuts can be taken at the stage to which the leaf-sheath of the lowest inter-node tends to separate. Care should be taken that the dry matter content of above 30% reduces the palatability in sorghum forage.

Bajra/Pearl Millet (*Pennisetum glaucum*)

Small millets or little millets or even lesser millets are widely grown in most of the Asian countries, Africa and Russia as a food crop. As such, in India, finger millet, little millet, barnyard millet, foxtail millet and spike millet are cultivated for grain and forage besides some new genotypes in Bajra (*Pennisetum typhoides*) have also been released for forage purposes only. Proso millet (*Panicum milaceum*) and foxtail millet (*Setaria italica*) are grown in Japan and Korea while broom corn (*Sorghum nervosum)* and foxtail millets are more popular. In South-east Russia, Proso millet and Broom corn are the most common but in USA, foxtail millet as a forage crop while Broom corn as a food crop are extensively cultivated.

Pearl millet is one of the most important grain and forage crop of agriculturally progressive area of India from Punjab, Haryana, U.P. and Bihar. It is native to tropical Africa and introduced into India before 2000 BC, has wide adaptability to grow well in saline to low pH soils as well as in low to high rainfall areas. It is one of the parentages of hybrid Napier is an annual fast growing 2.0 to 2.5m tall and erect with many tillers. Erectophyl flat leaves measures from 80 to 125 cm long and 2.5 to 3.5 cm wide. It bears very dense short panicles of 10 cm thick and upto 90 cm long. with short-pedicellated spikelets. The matured grains are covered with hairy-margin lemma and palea (Photo 1)

Package of Practices

About 5 kg seed/ha is sown in 40-45 cm in rows and 10-12 cm from seed to seed Basal application of 5-6 t FYM/ha with 20 kg N and 10-12 kg P/ha followed by 20 kg N/ha as top dressing after interculturing at one month is done. High pH soils usually deficient in Zn, application of 20 kg zinc sulphate/ha at tillering gives higher forage and grain yields. Cutting for forage can be taken after two months at 50% flowering.

Varieties

Some sufficient numbers of promising varieties of forage type bajra have been released for different regions of the country.

Varieties	Characteristics
Giant Bajra	It is developed by intervarietal hybridization between Australian and local bajra of Dhule (Maharashtra) followed by selections. Thin, high tillering, leafy and proteinous (CP 9-10%) and produces 60-75 t GF/ha is good for hay making. Resistant to diseases and cultivated in all the bajra growing areas.
Raj Bajra Chari-2	Developed after two cycles of full sib selection in population created through random mating among 20 crosses of 4 inbreds of west Africa. It is of medium yielding type (4o-45 t GF/ha) but resistant to all diseases. Internodes remain covered with leaf-sheath even at flowering is fit for growing else where.
CO-8	It is a hybrid of 732 A x Sweet Giant Bajra followed by pedigree selection. A low yielder (30 t GF/ha) in short period (50-55 days) but very soft and palatable, grown in south India.
APFB-2	Evolved by randomly mated population, is an early type, non-lodging, nutrient responsive for both summer and monsoon seasons is 160-180 cm tall with only 25 t GF/ha and 6 t DM/ha.
Proagro No.1 (FMH-3)	Produced from crossing of PSP 21 x PP-23. It gives 35 tGF/ha in single cut and 75 t/ha in multi-cut system within 90-95 days duration is recommended for entire country.
PCB-164	Selected from 5 late maturing lines is fit to grow in N-W India.
FBC-16	A multi-cut variety, resistant to major diseases with low oxalate concentration and voluntary dry matter eaten by animal is grown in north region, produces 70-80 t GF/ha.
Avika Bajra Chari (AVKB-19)	It is a selection made from local variety from Nagore (Rajasthan) It is of dual purpose and grown in N–W region, produces 35-37 t GF/ha and 8-9 t DM/ha as well as 10 t gain/ha.
Narendra Chari Bajra-2 (NDFB-2)	It is tolerant to salinity and suitable for problematic soils of north-east region (eastern U P and north Bihar).

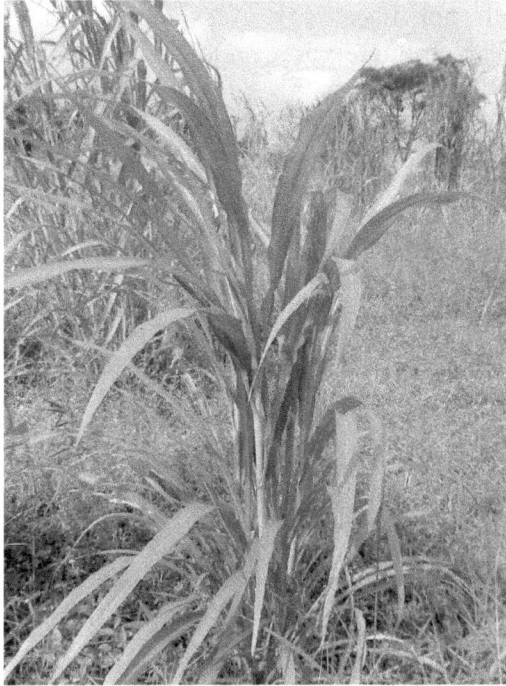

Photo1. Bajra (*Pennisetum glaucum* L.)

Teosinte/ Mak Chari (*Zea* sps.)

Teosinte or Mak Chari or Makhya bajra has four species (*Zea diploperennis, Z. perennis, Z. luxurians and Z. nicaraguensis*) belongs to Poaceae family is supposed to be the parent of maize. Plants are almost similar to maize , monoecious with male flower in a terminal called 'tussel' and female flowers at leaf axil with small 'ears'. It bears angular seeds of creamy white to deep brown in colours. Since, it is very easily crosses with maize accordingly, some new genotypes, known as 'Teomaize' has been developed for forage production in India. It is an annual cereal forage crop native to Central America. It grows up to a height of 3.5 m with smooth linear succulent leaves and stems. A well developed plant may have about 1.0m long leaves of 7-8 cm width. From America, it was imported to India in 1881and now cultivated in most of the maize growing areas of North India (Photo 2).

Varieties

Only a few varieties are available for cultivation *viz*; Improved Teosinte. It gives 35-45 t GF/ha under north and central zones while TL-1: It is tall type, profused tillering, leafy, of a little longer duration and free from leaf spot diseases. It gives more than 55 t GF/ha and 11 t DM/ha in Punjab and Haryana states.

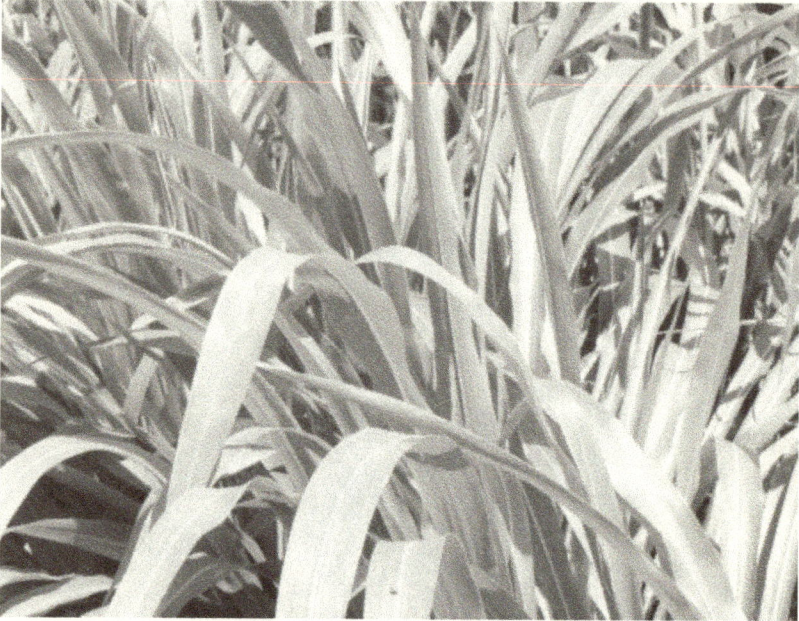

Photo 2. Teosinte (*Euchlena mexicana*)

Climate and Soils

Climatic requirement of teosinte is similar to maize as such hot-humid regions with average annual rainfall of 100-120cm followed by 28-35°C of temperature are conducive for its normal growth and development. Its water requirement is less than maize but higher than sorghum as such it also needs a well-drained sandy-loam to loam soils of medium fertility.

Cultural Operations

Since, it is a monsoonal or rainy season forage crop hence it is grown under rain-fed crop in India and if, the irrigation facility be at hand it can also be cultivated during summer season. It is sown either in rows or broadcast preferably with some legume like cowpea or soybean. Under drilled- row conditions, seeding at 40cm spacing 25-30 kg seeds/ha and for broadcast 40kg seeds/ha are used. Nutrients application in terms of 10 tonnes FYM/ha along with 25-30 kg N/ha, 30-35kg P_2O_5/ha and 25-30 kg K_2O/ha as basal followed by hoeing and weeding and top-dressing of 30-40 kg N/ha at one month crop gives a good forage yield to be cut after 80-90 days after sowing. Further application of 25-30 kg N /ha after the first cut can also give additional yield in second cut. Thus, a well managed crop can produce 40-50 tonnes of green forage/ha or 12-15 tonnes of dry matter/ha which contains about 8.5% of crude protein on dry weight basis. Among the few varities, Improved teosinte and TL-1 are usually cultivated in different states of North India.

For seeds production, June sown crop can be harvested in November. The harvested crop is usually left for 8-10 days to dry up before threshing. This way, 1.0-1.2tonnes seeds/ha can be available, can be grinded and fed to livestock or kept for sowing in next season.

Forage Maize (*Zea mays* L.)

Maize (Zea mays) belongs to family Poaceae is an important grain cereal and equally an important cereal forage crops grown through out the world. Among cereal forages it is the most nutritious and palatable at any stage of cutting and even after the harvest of cobs its quality is still far better than many cereals and grasses. In India, it covers about 1 million ha area. It is a fast growing plant and as a forage crop 5-6 crops can be taken in a year as it is cut after 55-60 days at 50% flowering or tussling.

Teosinte (*Zea perennis*) is supposed to be the parentage of maize (*Zea mays*) but it has no tillering habit. The stem of maize is thicker, soft and juicy than teosinte. Plant height of some of the varieties may be more than 300 cm tall with 20-30 long internodes and each node with strong leaf-sheath has 60-100 cm long and 5-10 cm broad leaf with very bold green mid rib. It bears male and female flowers seperatly of which male flowers appears few days earlier at the flag leaf than female which appears at one of the nodes, is fully covered with several layers of silks, known as cob. This cob has several female flowers of which each one is tagged with a tube known as pollen tubes. These tubes are responsible to accept the pollen and passes to ovary for fertilization and hence, formations of seeds take place.

Cultural Practices

Maize is known as a garden crop, meaning by it requires highly fertile soils. Recent alluvial to old alluvial soils with fine texture are the best soils for exploting its productivity. Soils with high pH (>7.5) and water logging are not desired. Though, it can be grown round the year but day and night temperatures below25°C and 15°C respectively, the growth is restricted. High humidity and medium rainfall and well-drained soil is essential.Under Indian conditions it is also sown during winter (December-January) as to harvest before April to avoid hot temperature of summer which results in to less seed formation or even complete male sterility and crop failure. Since a fine tilth is desired hence it needs good tilling.

Heavy composting with 20 t FYM/ha + 100-120 kg N/ha+ 25 kg P/ha+ 30 kg K/ha is applied.Basal application of compost + 1/4 to 1/3 N + full dose of P and K is done. Rest of N is applied as top dressing in two splits, first after interculturing at about 30 days of emergence and second at 45 days if it is to be cut for forage at 60-65 days. In case of seed production last dose of N is applied at flag leaf stage.

For forage production 40 kg seed/ha and for grain production 20 kg seed/ha is required. It is sown in rows with row to row and seed to seed distance at 40 cm x 15cm and at 75 cm x 20-25 cm for forage and seed production, respectively. As a summer crop 2-3 irrigations in a better water retaining capacity soils and 4-5 irrigations in low water retaining soils are applied.

Varieties	Characteristics
African Tall Composite	It is a composit of 7 genotypes (H-611 C, H-611, H-611 ®C3, K-11 x EC-573 (R12) C3, Ukkri compo A(F) C5 x Ukiri Comp A, (F) C3, Chitedge Comp A and Ilonga Comp developed through modified mass selection technique. Average 260 cm tall, more leafy and gives 60-70 t GF/ha and 3 t grain/ha. Grown through out the country is also resistant to diseases and moderately to borers.
ABFM-8	This is a synthetic variety derived from Varun (V-41) and Palampur local varietal cross advanced by mass selection. It is non-lodging, leafy of 180-200 cm tall bears orange grains matures in 90-100 days in kharif and 105-110 days in winter. Cutting at silking stage gives 345 t GF/ha and 7.5 t DM/ha is suitable for south India.
J-1006	This variety is released by crossing Makka safed 1-DR x Turpeno PB for northern states is very resistant to a number of diseases
Pratap Makka Chari-6	It is developed by compositing 11 early to medium white seeded entries is foud fit for growing in north-west part of the country. A medium tall type with bold stem and resistant to lodging, gives 45-50 t GF/ha at flowering and mature at 90-95 days.

Chapter 4
Tropical Forage Grasses

Cultivated Grasses

Deenanath Grass (*Pennisetum pedicellatum* Trin)

Deenanath Grass (India), Desho grass / Kyasuwa grass (Nigeria) belongs to family Poaceae, mostly annuals and a few perennials is native to both India (Jharkhand) and Nigeria. Now it is widly grown both as a cut-carry and as a pasture grass in several countries of Asia, Australia, Africa and US.

In India it was first identified and collected from forest areas of the then south Bihar (Jharkhand) round 1952 and first grown at Bihar Agricultural College, Sabour. Since it was first brought by Mr. Deenanath Jha hence it is known as Deenanath grass, name given by Chaterjee (1954) who first published a popular article in Indian Farming. Latter on it was brought to Ranchi and some very promising varieties (t_1, T3 and T15 and others) were developed through mass mating of which T15, the most popular one is still grown in different parts of the country.

It is an erect annual or perennial, 150-180 cm tall plant consisted of trilobed sterile lemma with 1-3 spikelets in clusters of which lower legule length is about half of spiklet. The spiklet cluster is subtended by involucres of 15-25 unfused bristles of 15-30 cm long with one very long.. Spiklet cluster is of 1 sessile and atleast I pedicellate spiklet which contain 1 each of fertile and sessile florate. Spiklets lanceolate, slightly dorsally compressed 3-4 mm long and 0.6-1.0 mm wide. Lower glume reduced, upper glume and sterile lemma as long as spikelet. Fertile lemma and palea coriaceous, glossy, translucent, fertile lemma 5 nerved. Caryopsis lanceolate, dorsally compresses, 0.5-2.5 mm long.

Package of Practices

It is sown during pre-monsoon or start of the monsoon in June-July. The field is cleaned and ploughed 2 times and after light plunking the seeds with fluffs @ 10-12 kg/ha or 2-2.5 kg seeds without fluffs are broadcasted followed by planking. It gives better results if sowing is done at 40 cm row to row spacing just below the soil not more than 2 cm deep. Transplanting of 5-6 weeks old seedlings is also preferred at 30 x 10 spacing It is very responsive to nutrient addition. Application of 5 t FYM and 20 kg N plus 10-12 kg P/ha followed by top dressing after 6 weeks in seed sown and after 2-3 weeks in planted crop gives a very good result. Generally application of K is avoided since its roots are efficient to change unavailable form of K into available form. At high fertility level an average of 3 years at 150 kg N/ha and 30 kg P_2O_5/ha, it produced 77.9 t GF/ha and 17.1 t DM/ha in alfisols of Ranchi (Bhagat *et al*, 1986). Earlier works of Mukherjee *et al.* (1981) and Narwal *et al.* also reported high response of this grass to N and P fertilization.

Initially crop growth is very slow but after interculturing of 5-6 week crop the growth is captured fastly. In forest areas or under silvipastoral system it is sown even without proper ploughing where crop is well established in the subsequent year by self seeding.

Varieties

In addition to old varieties some new promising varieties have been also released by the different institutes.

Varieties	Characteristics
T15	Developed through mass mating of local collection from Jharkhand forest and exotic genotypes from Nigeria. It is tall, drooping long leaves, with redish–brown colour at the lower internodes. Drooping or half curved panicle with long spike consisting of thinly placed seeds with redish brown colour which turned to brown at maturity. It gives 50-60 t GF/ha in two cuts and 70-75 t GF/ha when cut at 50% flowering with 20-25 % dry matter

Contd...

Varieties	Characteristics
Jawahar Pennisetum-12	The variety was derived from selection of strain from Pusa Bihar P.No. 12 by pedigree method by JNKVV, Jabalpur. It was recomnmended for cultivation in Madhya Pradesh in 1974. The variety is 156 cm tall, profused tillering (34/plant), the leaves are long and broad, with average leaf stem ratio of 1.27. It is suitable for two cutting systems, if 1st cut is taken at boot stage and second at 50% flowering the average green fodder production is 55-60 t/ha and 14 t DM/ha. .
Pusa Deenanath Grass:	The variety was developed through mass selection from African germplasm. The maturity period is 120-130 days and average green fodder production is 73 t/ha. The variety was released for cultivation for the entire country.
Bundel-1	The variety was developed through selection from indigenous collection from Madhya Pradesh has been notified for cultivation in entire country in 1987. It is a late maturing grass with purple stem. There are abundant long velvet hairs on ventral surface of the leaf. The spike is very large and loose. The large spikelets have long bristles. The variety yields 30-40 t/ha green fodder. The plants have high field resistance to leaf spots.
Bundle-2	The variety was released through pedigree selection of IGFRI 3808-4-2-1. The variety has been notified for cultivation in entire country. This is a late maturing. purple stemmed having abundant long velvet hairs on ventral surface of the leaf. It has very large loose spike. Large spikelets with long bristles. The average yield is 48 t/ha. It has high tolerance to leaf spot. Helminthosporium and other major diseases and insect pests, is resistance to lodging drought hardy and is high fertilizer responsive.
COD-1	The variety was developed through gamma radiation (30 KR) mutation of Dinanath T 3 and released in 1995. This variety has been recommended for cultivation in Tamil Nadu under rainfed as well as irrigated conditions. It closely resembles like T3. The green fodder yield is 40-50t/ha.

In addition to annual types, 'Agros-4" a perennial type developed at Ranchi gave more than 200 t green herbage/ha under long duration monsoon of Kerala and Andman- Nicobar islands.

Hybrid Napier (*Pennisem purpureum* Schum.)

Napier grass is a robust-tufted perennial. The genus *Pennisetum* has more than 60 annuals and perennials cereals as well as grasses grown in tropical to sub-tropical countries of Asia, Africa, USA and Southern European continents. Flat (4-5cm) and long (1.0-1.2 m) erectophyl leaves, Stem resembles like to that of sugarcane but relatively with swollen at the nodes followed by rudimentary auricle. A fully grown plant may be as long as 3-4m having thickness of 1.0-3.5 cm diameter. Inflorescence is spike-like panicle with compact or in groups of sterile branchlets.

A vigorus, hardy, high yielding perennial grass is native to South Africa which derived its name from Colonel Napier, who first drew the attention of the then Rhodesian presently Zimbabwe Government in 1909 as a forage crop, as such it bears his name. Secondly, since, even the elephants roaming inside the forest of this species are hidden from the view hence, it is also known as elephant grass.

Since, the original Napier grass was less in productivity as well as in quality hence, the attempts were made to bring an improvement in yield and quality. Therefore, Burton (1944) crossed Bajra (*Pennisetum typhoides*) with Napier (*Pennisetum purpureum*) and evolved the species known as Hybrid Napier or Giant Napier or Napier x Bajara Hybrid but it failed to get recognition as the desirable characteristics were not recorded. In 1951 N. Krishnaswami also evolved a Napier x Bajra hybrid but this was also not accepted. Again, Burton (1965) tried and succeeded in developing a new hybrid and received recognition all over the world. However, the flowers of the Hybrid Napier failed to bear fertile seeds due to male sterility and therefore, it is a vegetitavelly propagated. In India, Gupta (1974) released a number of hybrid varieties of which 'Gajraj' was the first one with 12% more yield than Napier. He further evolved 'NB 21' with 40% higher yield than original Napier. There after a large number of Hybrids were released to grow under different agro-climatic conditions.

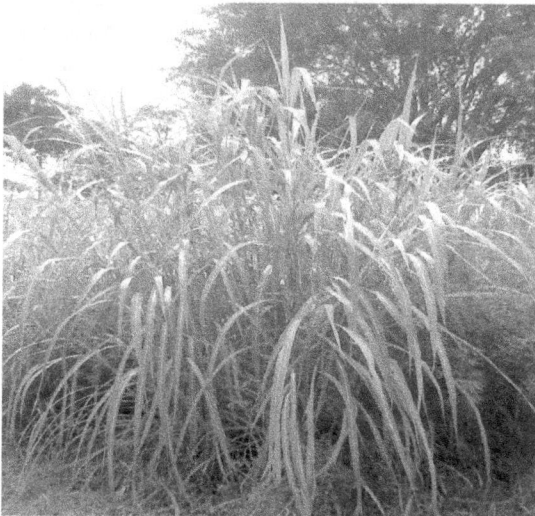

Photo 3. Hybrid Napier

These varieties are vigorous in character with more succulent, long and flat leaves, tall plant types with profused tillering and fast regeneration capacity under multi-cut system. Besides, 2.0 to 2.5 time higher production potential to simple Napier, it is also relatively more nutritious (Photo 3).

Climate and Soils

Hybrid Napier favours hot and humid climate to exploit its full yield potential but it can be extended up to a sub-tropical conditions. It can sustain well under 30 to 40°C but maximum yield can be harvested at temperature between 30-35°C. It remains dormant at temperature below 15°C. It usually suffers from cold injury and thus temperature below 4°C is injurious to survive. It is well cultivated from 25°N to 20°S latitudes from sea level to1500m altitude. As the elevation, increased, the yields are also reduced, accordingly. An annual rain fall between 1200- 1500mm is required but it can also be produced during hot season if, irrigation facility be at hand. It requires wide range of sandy-loam to clay-loam vertisols with good fertile well-drained soils of slightly acidic to slightly alkaline (pH 5.7 to 7.5) in reaction.

Cultural Practices

Being the highest yield potential forage crop, it requires deep ploughing for the development of its well developed root system which in turn results in the maximum bio-mass out come. Therefore, one deep ploughing with soil turning plough followed by 2 with cultivators and finally planking is required. Application of well rotten compost or FYM @15-20 tonnes/ha can be thoroughly mixed with 25-30 kg N/ha + 40kg P_2O_5/ha and 30-40 kg K_2O/ha at the time of planting the cuttings is done. For planting, stems cuttings or rooted slips can be cut in pieces consisted of 3 nodes. Furrows can be made at 50-60 cm apart for sole crop and at 1.0-2.0 m for intercropping or for moving of the power tillers/ tractors for cultural practices and sowing of annual forages. Thus, for pure Napier grass planting at row to row and plan to plant distances of 50 cm for both sides can be kept which, will require just 40,000 sets/ha where as for intercropping number of sets can be less as per rows distances but plant to plant spacing will be the same. These sets are planted by putting one node below the soil surface, the middle one just above touching the soil surface while, top third one in the air or above the ground making an angle of 45° from the soil surface. Flat planting by putting some soil at the middle node is also done. It is better to plant this grass during monsoon period or just after winter month as summer forage under irrigated conditions. Growing Napier grass, particularly in acid soils, requires some insecticides during planting to protect the crop from termites etc. Therefore, application of 20-25 kg 5%Aldrin dust at planting as well as in subsequent years at the start of rain should be done.

As the grass is progressing, 2 inter-culturing and weeding may be done. Since, the grass has potential to produce the highest yield among several other forages hence, it requires high level of nutrients. As such, besides basal application of nutrients, addition of 40kgN/ha at one month crop as well as after each cut, gives the desire yields. In absence of nitrogenous fertilizer for top-dressing, application of poultry litters @ 4-5 tonnes/ha or combination of 20-25 kg N/ha + 2-3 tonnes poultry litters/ha, gives a wonder full harvest of the green herbage. Among the 3 promising varieties (NB21, IGFRI-6 and HGN/BN-1) tested, IGFRI-6 produced significantly the maximum green forage (74.4 t/ha) and dry of matter (12.8 t/ha) yields in 3 cuts at 60 kg N/ha/cut(Prasad and Kumar, 1995).

Cutting Management

In the establishment year, first cutting is taken after 8-10 weeks of planting and subsequently at 6 weeks interval at a plants height of preferably 80-100 cm by leaving 8-10 cm from the ground surface. This way from second year onwards, 60-70 tonnes/ha of green forage or 15-20 tonnes dry matter/ha in 3 cuttings can be taken. If, irrigations are provided during the summer months, altogether 5-6 cuttings can give 120-150 tonnes green or 30-40 tonnes dry matter/ha.

Growth of this perennial is restricted in cold season when temperature fall bellow 15°C. Under such situations, sowing of Lucerne or Berseem can be done to utilize the production from the same land under irrigated condition. It requires a basal dressing of nutrients once in a year preferably at or just before the onset of monsoon @ 10-15 tonnes FYM/ha+40kg n/ha + 40 kg P_2O_5/ha+30 kg K_2O/ha. It gives maximum yields during second and third years of planting. There after, the yield is reduced in succeeding years due to fall in soil fertility which can be controlled by mixing or intercropping of legumes to some extent. It is advised to change the plot after 3-4 years.

Nutritive Value

Though, Hybrid Napier is the highest herbage producing forage crop however, it is of less nutritive values. On an average it contains about 8-10% CP hence, it is recommended to grow it with legumes. In tropics, sowing of either Cowpea/Kudzu/Soybean in rainy season followed by Lucerne / Clover/ *Desmodium* spps. in winter within the grass as a mixed or intercrop, provides extra forages as well as balance ration besides, it maintains the soil fertility. As such, intercropping of cowpea in Kharif season and Berseem in Rabi season within 1.0m row spacing of Hybrid Napier with use of 30kgN/ha/cut in acid Alfisols, was recorded an improvement in yield and quality of the forages along with the maximum net returns (Bhagat, *et al.*, 1992).

Varieties

Sufficient numbers of high yielding hybrid varieties have been released by different Agricultual universities and ICAR institutes during last over three decades.

Varieties	Characteristics
CO-1	This variety a cross of Bajra x Napier (Merkeson) is tolerant to drought.It attends 230 cm height, non-lodging, high tillering (26 tillers/culm) leafy (354 leaves/culms) with high L:S ratio (0.94) and has black purple panickle. It is grown in south region of India in which 300 t GF/ha is obtained. Later on 2 more varieties CO-2 and CO-3 were developed but their yields were very less than CO-1
Hybrid Napier-3 (Swetika)	Crossing of Napier grass x Bajra (PSB-2) gives birth of this variety which is erect, profused tillering, narrow upright leaves in thin stems has fast regenerating capacity. It is resistant to acid soils and gives 70-80 t GF/ha and 18 t DM/ha in central India.
Yashwant(RBN-9)	It is evolved through hybridization of Giant Bajra x Napier grass and grown in irrigated area of Maharastra. It gives 150 t GF/ha. with 10% protein and only 2.4% oxalic acid.
IGFRI-5	It is drought resistant and cultivated in Himachal Pradesh below 800m elevation. A vigorous tall growing with thin tillers and very leafy (14-15 leaves/tiller), glabrous and soft stems gives 100-115 t GF/ha and 35-37 t DM/ha with 6% protein and 2.8% oxalate.. Another IGFRI-6 variety is also found suitable for acid soils.
NB-21	A fast growing with profused tillering with non-hairy stems and long-narrow smooth leaf blade.
NB-37	Dwarf hybrid for sub-tropic pasture and wastelands of zone I and II of HP that gives only 35-40 t GF/ha

Contd...

Varieties	Characteristics
PBN 233	It is through hybridization of Bajra composit 1 x N-23 (Napier). It provides very high yield of forage round the year in Punjab (375 t GF/ha) is a photosensitive and flowers only in winter like NB-21 and PBN-83.
KKM-1	Developed from crossiong of Bajra-IP 1507 x Napier FD 429 followed by clonal selection is leafy and high tillering, grown in southern Tamil Nadu which produces 250 t GF/ha
APBN-1	A cross of IPM-12 159 (Nigeria) x elephant grass is medium tall (70 cm) produces 50 tillers/club with deep green leaves, gives very high yield (200t GF/ha) in Gujarat.
Suguna	It is also a very high yielding semi-perennial variety (260 t GF/ha) for Kerala obtained from the cross of Composite 9 x FD 431 followed by clonal selection.
Supriya	It is like Suguna with almost similar yield potential (270 t GF/ha) has been developed from crossing of TNSC 4 x FD 471followed by clonal selection.
Sampoorna (DHN 6)	A hybrid of IPM 14188 (Bajra line) x FD 184 (Napier line) followed by clonal selection is good for Karnataka under irrigated conditions. It has low oxalate content (2%) and gives 120-150 t GF/ha in 6-8 cuts.

Job's Tear (Coix)

Coix (*Coix lacryma jobi* blad Linn.) belongs to family Poaceae is resistant to high moisture condition but not enough resistant to water logging to that of Para grass (*Brachiaria mutica*). It has more diversity in Indo-china – Indonesia and is tolerant to low pH lateritic soils.

Robust annuals of 100-300 cm tall branched culms, loose sheath, teret, striate, glabrous ligule (1.5-2.0 cm long), margins erose and minutely fringed blades 10-50 cm long, 20-50 cm wide, glabrous or coarse. Inflorescences numerous, terminal and axillary, each consisting of separate pistilate and staminate racemes, cupules borne on long stout peduncle from axis of upper leaves, white or bluish, bony, lustrous, globose-ovoid, 5-15 cm long.

Cultural Practices

It is grown in tropical conditions of rice growing areas under rainfed conditions. Propagated either through dribbling or broadcasting of seeds (10-15 kg/ha) during onset of monsoon. Its cultivation is very limited and grown only in North-East region of high rainfall areas.

Varieties

KCA-3, KCA-4 and Bidhan Coix-1 are the few varieties which are released by BCKV, Kalyani, recently. Among these, last one is more promising that gives about 35 t /GF/ha, 7.0 t DM/ha.

Pasture/Range Grasses

Thin Napier grass (*Pennisetum polystachyon* Sch.)

Thin Napier or Mission grass belongs to genus *Pennisetum*, is a perennial with thin stem as compared to Napier is a drought resistant grass. It grows with a plant height from 1.5 -2.0 m with light green medium pointed leaves at the apex. These leaves are fully covered with small fluffs on dorsal as well as on ventral sides. In winter season, the upper portion of the leaves turns to reddish-brown but not as deep as to the leaves of perennial Deenanath grass (*P. pedecellatum*). The panicles resemble like perennial Deenanath grass but comparatively thin and long with yellowish in colour is more succulent and soft than other range grasses (Photo 4).

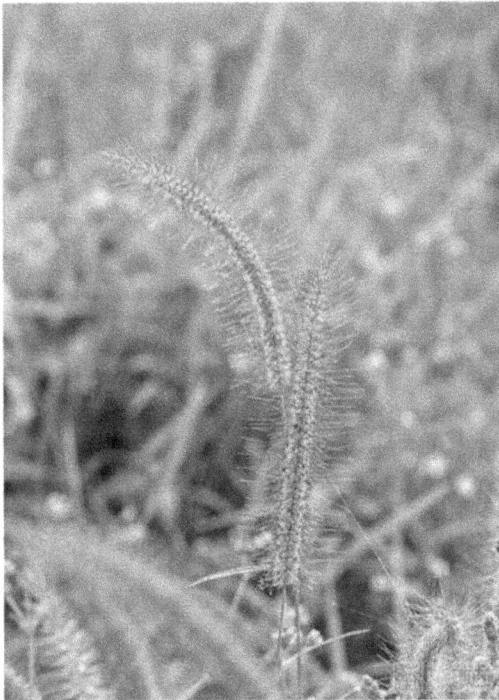

Photo 4. Thin Napier Grass / Mission Grass (*P. polystachyon* Sch.)

Soils and Climate

It performs well in sandy-loam soils with good drainage system as well as it is successfully grown in laterite acidic soils of high rainfall areas having low water retaining capacity to alkaline semi-arid soils of low rain receiving regions. However, high temperature, high humidity and high rainfall coastal upland soils are the best suited conditions for its yield maximization. Similar to Napier grass, temperature below 15°C is injurious for its growth.

Cultural Practices

Thin Napier has profuse seed production potential and therefore, it is propagated through seeds as well as rooted culms. These seeds are even smaller than the seeds of annual *P. pedicellatum* hence, it is sown just 1-2 cm deep into the soil. Two ploughings with cultivators and leveling is enough for sowing or transplanting of the rooted culms. It may also be sown as broad-caste in rangelands with clay soils pellets by air dropping. Under well managed cultivated conditions, only 2-3 kg seed/ha without fluffs is required while, 7-8 kg seeds/ha with fluffs is sufficient. Composting with 8-10 tonnes FYM/ha at sowing can give a good stand. Application of 30-40 kg N/ha after establishment of the grass as well as after each cutting gives a better bio-mass yields. Since, Thin Napier grass and *Stylosanthes guianensis* var. Schofield or Graham are equally competitive hence, intercropping of grass and legume in alternate rows with full seed rates of the both species is suggested for higher and balance forage production.

Cutting Management and Yields

If, the grass is sown or transplanted during mid June, first cutting can be taken in last week of August and second cut in mid October but from second year and onward, cutting can be taken at an interval of 5-6 weeks. This way 50-60 tonnes green herbage/ha/yr with 22-25% dry matter and 7-8% CP can be obtained. As per one report of the Forest Department, this grass is very much like by the elephants in Eastern Indian states. This grass is very quick in establishment and has well developed root system to protect the soils from water erosion and gives a very good strength to bunds in canal areas.

Gamba grass (*Andropogan gayanus* Linn.)

Genus *Andropogon* has the two important palatable perennial grass species; *Andropogon gayanus* and *A. pumilus*. Since, the first one can sustain under hot and dry conditions of the summer and even remains green hence, it is also known as "Sadabahar grass", meaning ever green (Chatterji, 1970). It is a very thin-stemmed of 2.5-3.0 cm fully grown plant. Leaf sheath and entire leaf are fully covered with small whitish hairs. About one third lower portion of the leaf is cylindrical or say petiolated. Leaves are as long as 80- 100 cm with 2-3 cm broad but it may be short and thin during summer months. In winter season, margin and upper parts of the leaves turn to brownish-red colour, known as winter injury.The flowers are very small on the spike of spiklets which, appear on few upper most nodes. The plants of other species are more leafy without hairs but a little more hard than the first one (Photo 5).

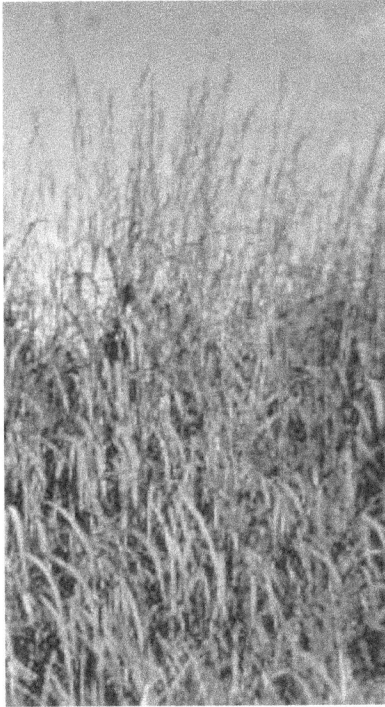

Photo 5. Sadabahar Grass / Gamba Grass *(Andropogan gayanus)*

Soils and Climates

It is widely grown in red acid soils of South America, India, Australia and Africa. This grass is very draught resistant and recommended as one of the best grass for pasture production. It requires low fertile soils as such available phosphorus requirement is the lowest (2.5ppm) among several range and pasture species. Though, it gives a bumper harvest under high humidity, high temperature and rainfall conditions however, it also sustains in low rainfall and high temperature in semi-arid regions.

Cultural Practices

It is treated as a cultivated as well as an ideal pasture and range grass of low to high rainfall areas of low moisture retaining soils. It is generally propagated through rooted slips since 25-30 percent seeds are only viable. For pure stand, row to row and plant to plant distance at 70 cm and 50 cm are kept, respectively. As associated grass, with legume like, *Stylosanthes* spps. or *Arachis glabreta*, at row to row distance of 100 cm can be maintained and either of the legume can be sown between the rows. In low to medium fertile soils, basal application of 20 kg N/ha and equal amount of P_2O_5 can be sufficient. However as a mixed stand with legume, addition of only phosphorus will be sufficient. After 5-6 weeks one weeding should be done.

Cutting Management and Yield

Grass established from rooted slips, first cutting after 8 weeks and subsequent cuts after each 6 weeks can be taken. In the second year, 70-80 tones green forage/ha in 3 cutting can be obtained while, from succeeding years onwards 50-60 tonnes green forage/ha with 25-27% dry matter and 6-7% CP can be harvested (Prasad and Prasad, 1982). Application of 30-40 kg N/ha after each cuts gives higher bio-mass. As a pasture grass its regeneration capacity is very fast and under seepage conditions, it is still very fast (Prasad and Prasad, 1977).

Brachiaria sps

Genus *Brachiaria* is a large genus of over 120 species of both annual and perennial grown in tropics and sub-tropical climates of the world. Presently, Para grass (*Brachiaria mutica*) an ideal grass for water-logged conditions while, Paladide grass (*B. brizantha*) and Signal grass (*B. decumbens*) as a drought resistant grass, are suitable for pasture and rangeland conditions.

Para Grass (Brachiaria mutica Stapf.)

Para Grass (*B. mutica* Stapf.) of Posaseae family is a perennial runner, profusely rooted at the nodes is a coarse type with full of puffs on the leaf, leaf-sheath and nodes. The length of runners may be from 2 to 5 meters, if frequent cuttings are not taken. Hollow stems facilitate to float on the water surface and as a resistant to water-logging. It bears deep green 20-25 cm long and 1.5-2.5 cm broad pointed leaves. The inflorescence is consisted of 3-5 sub-rachis with flowers hanging on the lower sides (Photo 6).

History and Distribution

Para Grass is native to Brazil from where it was introduced to different tropical countries including India around 1894 in Pune and now it is grown in almost all parts of India in general and dairy farms of coastal regions in particular.

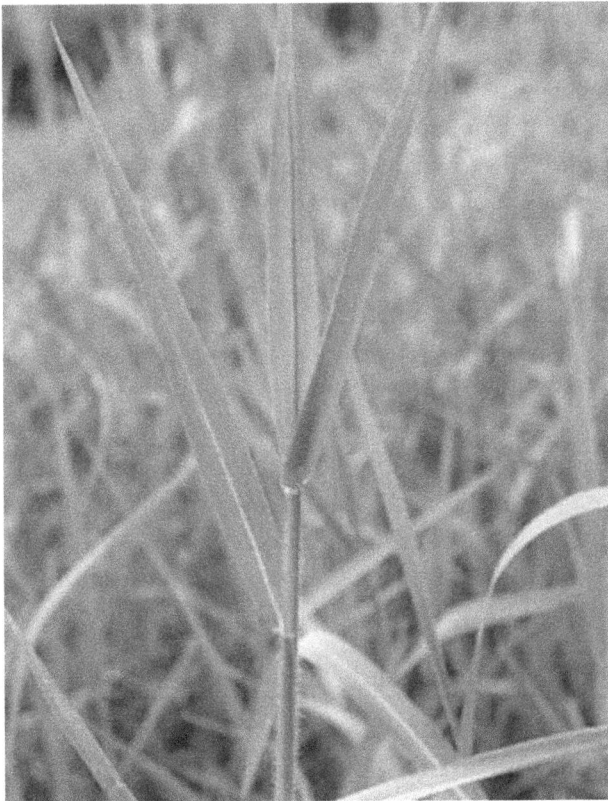

Photo 6. Para Grass (*Brachiaria mutica*)

Soils and Climate

This grass performed very well in water-logged soils with very wide pH range, from extremely acid soils to medium alkaline as well as in saline soils. It is also resistant to iron toxicity in acid soils. Its production potential under dairy seepage conditions is very out standing. Being a tropical grass, it requires high temperature, high humidity and high rainfall. It can also be cultivated in summer months at temperature above 40°C under irrigated conditions. It is also usually grown on ponds and canal bunds and marshy lands where there is no any option to grow any other crops except deep water paddy.

Cultural Operations

A very low percentage of viable seeds are produced by this grass therefore, it is multiplied through stem cuttings. Stems are cut by keeping 3 nodes and are planted on ridges at row to row and plant to plant spacing of 50-60 cm each.

Among the 3 nodes, one is kept below the soil surface at 45° inclination. As it is usually grown in low land or under dairy seepage conditions or along the bunds of lakes and ponds hence, hardly any nutrient is applied. If sown in flat upland soils, frequent irrigation and basal dressing of 15-20 tonnes compost/ha. and top dressing of 30-40 kg N/ha gives a better herbage yield.

Cutting Management and Yields

The first cutting of grass may be taken after 80-90 days of planting and depending on the plant growth, succeeding cuts may be possible at an interval of 4-6 weeks. Under normal conditions, green forage yield of 100-125 tonnes/ha can be harvested but under dairy seepage conditions it is one of the highest biomass producer with 250-275 tonnes green herbage/ha in 6-8 cuts/year. It contains 18-20% dry matter and 6-7% CP on green weight basis. In some of the countries it is also managed as a pasture grass but in India it is grown as a cut forages.

Signal grass (B. decumbens) and Palisade grass (B. brizantha)

These two species of genus *Brachiaria* are almost similar in morphological characteristics. Both perennials are of semi-erect type with leaves of Signal grass are comparatively more broad and green as compared to Palaside grass as well as the former is a more running and anchoring to soils hence, it is also used to give a good strength to the bunds. The 20-25 cm long leaves are very pointed at the tips. The inflorescence with 3-5 sub-rachis placed parallel to the ground surface and looks like train signal hence, the name is given as such (Photo 7).

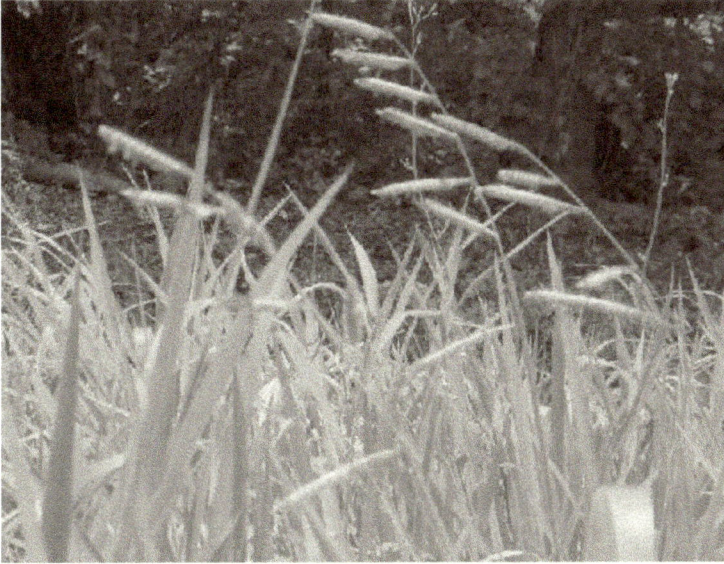

Photo 7. Signal grass (*B. decumbens*)

Soils and Climates

These grasses are very ideal for pasture production in acid soils since, among the two; Signal grass is the most resistant to aluminium and iron toxicity. The phosphorus requirement is also very low which enable it to grow successfully in such soils deficient in available-P. As these are the draught resistant grass hence, can be planted in semi-arid areas and high rainfall areas where, moisture holding capacity of the soils is very low (<25-30%) for pasture production.

Cutting/Grazing

Similar to Para grass, first cutting or grazing can be allowed after 8 weeks of planting and depending on growth and height, the subsequent cutting/grazing may be allowed after a gap of 4-6 weeks. Signal grass is well sustained to grazing due to an excellent root system well anchoring to soils, difficult to be up-rooted by the animals. Under cut and carry system with 40kgN/ha/cut, it gave about 80 tones of green herbage in 4 cuts taken at an interval of 6 weeks in second year but yield reduced to 40-50 tones/ha in subsequent years (Prasad *et al.*, 1982).

Guinea Grass (*Panicum maximum* Jacq.)

Genus, *Panicum* Linn.belongs to a very large genus consisted of above 500 species of annual and perennial grasses and food crops around the tropical to temperate countries of the world. It is a tall, erect with several rhizomes which give birth to daughter plants. Plant height of above 2.5m may attend under favourable weather conditions having hairy nodes and leaves up to 75cm long and 3-4cm flat with panic margins which turn to more sharp at maturity hence, the name Panicum is given. The inflorescence is divided in to multi-sub-branches and in whorls of spikelets in which seeds are covered with lemma and palea (Photo 8).

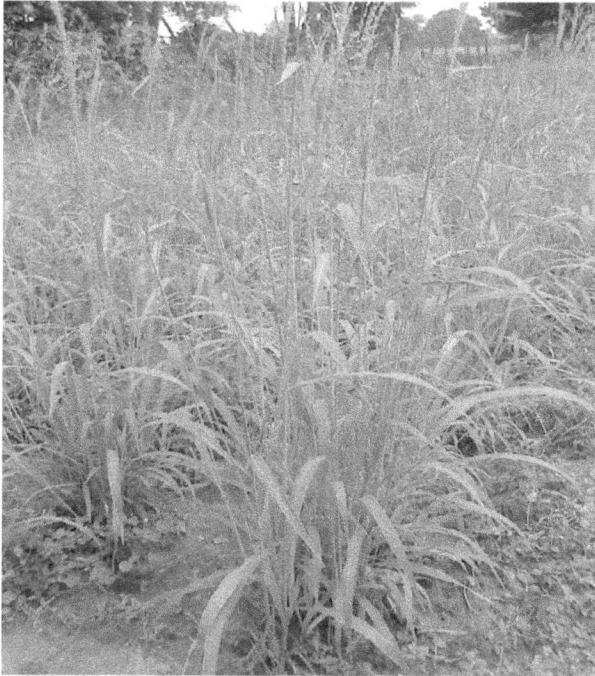

Photo 8. Guinea Grass (*Panicum maximum* Jacq.)

Origin and History

Guinea Grass (*Panicum maximum*) and Blue Panic Grass (*Panicum antidotale*) are the two important grasses of genus *Panicum*. The first one is a tropical species while the other one is temperate. Probably Guinea grass is native to tropical Africa and introduced to India as early as in 1793 and became the oldest among the imported grasses. It is widely grown as a dominating pasture grass in Australia, southern America and many islands like Philippines. In India, now adays, it has become a dominant grass under the Silvi-pasture system.

Climate and Soils

Guinea grass is well sustained from high intensity radiant energy to shade conditions. Therefore, it is the most ideal grass for Silvi-pasture system. This is one of the two grasses including *Brachiaria species* of which roots, the nodules containing N-fixing bacteria were isolated. Probably these bacteria prefer shade conditions for their development hence, grasses grown under the shades of trees are greener than those grown as sole crop in open fields. Though, it favours hot and humid climate with high rainfall but it is also successfully grown during hot summer months under irrigated conditions. It is very resistant to soil acidity and sustained well under the toxic levels of iron and aluminium in the soils. Light to medium loam soils without water logging is fit for this fast growing forage species.

Package of Practices

This grass produces very high number of seeds hence, it is propagated from seeds as well as from rooted slips. Though, synchronization in maturity of the seeds are absent even though sufficient number of viable seeds are available for sowing and maintaining a good plant population. About 2-3 kg seeds/ha is sufficient for sowing in 40-50 cm row spacing. The rooted slips are planted at row to row and plant to plant distances of 60cm and 40cm, respectively. Under rainfed or for pasture system, sowing is done before the onset of monsoon. For irrigated forage, February or early March sowing is preferred to get green herbage cut in summer months and the same continued in rainy season till the arrival of winter. One inter-culturing and weeding is done after 40-45 days of sowing/planting. Addition of FYM with some amount of inorganic source of nutrients gives fast cutting and high yield due to more number of cuttings. Therefore, basal application of 10-20tonns FYM/ha followed by top dressing of 30-40kg N/ha after weeding and hoeing and also after each cut gives a very good result. In 8-10 cuttings/year, 100-125 tonnes/ha green herbage with 20-25% dry matter and 6.5-7.5%CP can be harvested. Hamil and Macuenni are grown in south India while PGG-1 and PGG-9 and PGG-19 are some of the newly developed genotypes from Punjab, gave more yield over the traditional one in north India.

Varieties

A large number of varieties have been developed by different Agricultual Universities of the country for growing in their respective areas.

Varieties	Characteristics
Macueni	It is an exotic variety, leaves with full of hairs, erect, tufted and drooping as it becomes older. This has performed well in Kerala with 70-80 t GF/ha
Riversdate	It is also introduced in Kerala under the Indo-Swiss project and is suitable for growing in south India which gives about 75 t GF/ha.
Hamil	It is a very luxerant growth type and grown in all the hot- humid and acid soils of the country from Kerala, eastern coast to N-E and Jharkhand states.
Haritha and Marathakam	Both varieties are developed through mutation of F.R. 600, for south part of the country attends 175 cm of height in 6 months and medium yielder (55 t GF/ha).
Harthasree	A selection from JHGG 96-4 is good for growing in upland of Kerala
CO-1	A selection from Coimbatore local has a very high yield potential (200 t GF/ha is identified with serrated ventral surface lamina.
CO -2	A cross of CO-1 x Centenario is good for multi-cut and is grown in TN as perennial forage under irrigated conditions. It is resistant to lodging, shade loving with 80-100 tillers/clump, attends 250-270 cm height, very leafy and gives upto 270 t GF/ha/year.
Punjab Guinea Grass 1	Introduced from Australia (CPI 59985) is fit for N-W and hill zone which matures in 7 months.
PGG 9	It is an obligateapomictic from a cross between a sexual clone 82059 and obligate apomictic clone 80013 which has long, broad light green leaves with thick stem. Compact panicle with synchronic flowering and seed settimg. It gives 45-50 t GF/ha in 2 cttings containing 8-10% protein is suited for wastelands of Punjab state.
PGG 19	It is a hybrid of CPI 63450 (sexual line) x CPI 60013 (apomictic line) and selection of the obligate apomictic plants. It gives about 100 t GF/ha and 18\17-18 t DM/ha in 4 cuts is grown in Punjab.
PGG 14	A hybrid with profused tillering with leaf sheath more hairy than Hamil with 90 t GF/ha is grown in central zone of low rainfall area.
PGG 101	It is also a hybrid variety late flowering with bold seeds
PGG 518	A cross of clone P_5 and PGG-9 (male). It is grown under irrigated conditions in summer, late flowering with high yield potential of about122 t GF/ha in frequent cuts at an interval of 4-5 weeks.
PGG 616	Developed from the cross between a sexual clone of P-5 and PGG-101 is alike to PGG 518 except that more proteinous (11%) but low yield (47 t GF/ha).
Bundel Guinea-1 (JHGG-96-5)	Developed through selection from TGPM 19 (IG10-80) has glabrous leaf with thick stem is grown round the year in almost all parts of the country under irrigated conditions and claimed for high protein content (13.3 %) or more than several cereals grain crops.
Bundel Guinea-2 (JHGG 04-01)	It is for rainfed area with an yield of 50-60 t GF/ha and 15-18 t DM/ha.

Blue Panic Grass (*Panicum antidotale* Retz.)

Blue Panic Grass is also known as Australian drought resistant grass is an erect perennial to a height of 125-150cm. It is deep rooted, thin stemmed with distinct nodes and blue deep colour leaves of 40-45cm long and about 1cm width. It bears terminal pyramidal loose branched inflorescence with drooping spikelets on the sub-rachis.

Origin and History

Though, this grass was found in wild form in sub-desert area of Rajasthan but it was not recognized as a forage species until and unless it got forage value by the Australians. Since, it is the most drought resistant grass hence, it is found in association with xerophytic shrubs. Besides its adaptability in arid and semi-arid regions, it is also found around Nilgiri hills of Karnataka under sub-temperate conditions.

Soils and Climates

It is grown from light sandy to clay soils of neutral to slightly alkaline as well as in saline soils. As it is suitable for drought as well as under low temperature conditions, it is grown in low to high elevations having annual rainfall even less than 150mm.

Package of Practices

It is an ideal grass for pasture and rangeland conditions in arid and semiarid regions. If necessary, one light harrowing is enough for surface sowing of the very small seeds. In some areas, it is also raised through seedlings as a transplanted grass. Application of nutrients through fertilizers is usually not done but some manuring is done for proper establishment. Though, grazing is preferred at early age of the grass but as a cut forage 4-5 cuts at an interval of 6-8 weeks or before flag leaf initiation may give 20-25 tonnes green herbage/ha with 25-30% dry matter which contains about 6.5% CP.

Setaria sps.

The genus *Setaria* is consisted of two popular forage species; *Setaria sphaceolata* and *Setaria anceps*. The first one is known as Kazugula grass. Both are perennial types. Among the different perennial grasses, *S. sphacelata* is more succulent and nutritious with flattend stems similar to Ragi (*Eleusine coracana*) which is grown as a grain as well as a forage crop. The leaves are 30-40cm in length and 8-12cm in width with tightly attached leaf-sheath over the internode. These leaf sheaths turn to brown-red in colour under low temperature of winter months. The panicle is thin and compact as compared to the panicles of *Pennisetum spps.* In early stage it is of yellowish colour which turns to purple at maturity (Photo 9).

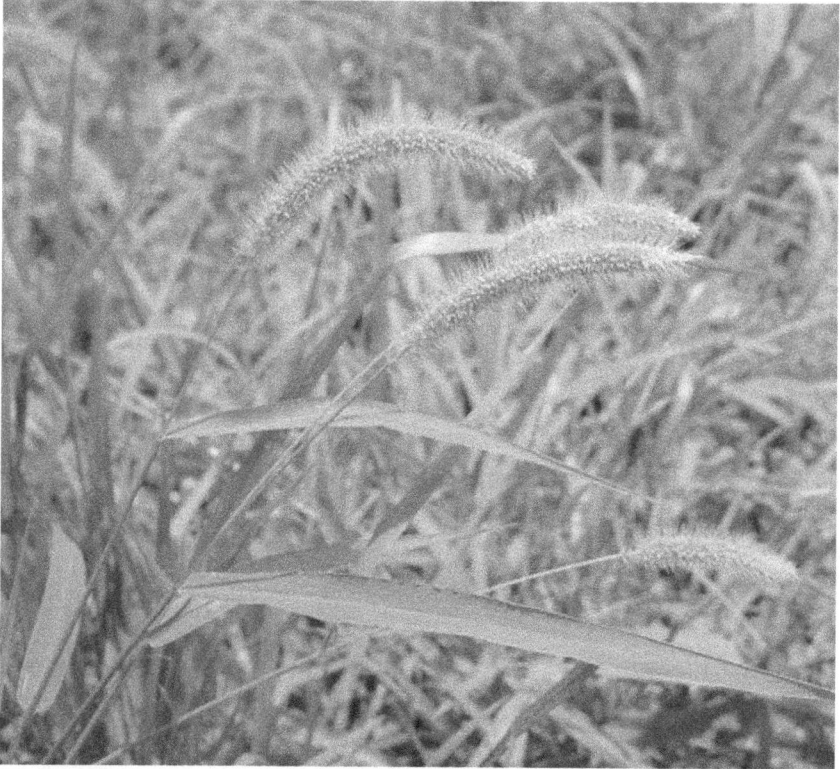

Photo 9. *Setaria sphaceolata*

Soils and Climate

Its performance in well fertilized soils is outstanding. Fertile sandy-loam to loam soils from medium acidity to neutral is better for its normal production. It is one of the fastest regenerating grasses grown under seepage conditions in summer months (Prasad and Prasad, 1977) in acid soils. High rainfall area having annual rainfall of above 1500mm is favourable for this grass.

Varieties

Some of the varieties are developed at Palampur (H.P., India) for sub-tropical regions of the country.

Varieties	Characteristics
Nandi	It is a fast growing and fast re-generating variety as well. Flat succulent stem with dark greenish yellow leaves and compact panicle bearind seeds with tiny flufs. It provides forage except in winter months (December-January and very responsive to nutrients and sewage water irrtgations. In 5-6 cuts at an interval of 5-6 weeks it gives 70-80 t GF/ha and contains 7-8 % protein.
PSS 1 (Golden timody	It is a selection from Narok-5, a Kenyan genotype for cultivation in sub-tropical uplands (1100-2100 m altitude). It is of thick stems with brown rusty head. It is cold resistant and provides green herbage except slow growth in wointer months. In 3-4 cuts 50-60 t GF/ha with 10% protein and low oxalates content (2-3%).
Setaria 92	It is for relatively low latitude pastures of the hilly low lands with low yield potential of 30 t GF/ha and about 7 t DM/ha in 1-2 cuttings.

Package of Practices

This grass requires relatively a better land preparation than other perennials. One ploughing with soil turning plough followed by two with cultivators and planking can be optimum for transplanting of the rooted slips. Though, this produces sufficient quantity of seeds but their germination percentage is very low. Planting can be done in rainy season and also in spring season under irrigated conditions to get green herbages during summer months. Application of 10-12 tonnes FYM/ha with 20-25 kg N/ha, 30-40kg P_2O_5/ha and 25-30kgK_2O/ha at planting followed by top-dressing of 30-40kgN/ha after 4 weeks of planting gives a good result. The grass can be cut after 8-10 weeks of planting and subsequently after 5-6 weeks intervals .Top-dressing of 25-30kgN/ha after alternate cutting gives 8-10 tonnes of fresh forage/ha which contains about 18-20% dry matter and 8-10% CP on green weight basis.

Since, the grass is fairly resistant to low temperature hence, it make possible to harvest some yield in winter months also. It is fit for as cut forage, silage, hay as well as for grazing purposes. Besides Nandi and Kazungula, Narok and PSS-1 are some of the other promising varities, cultivated under sub-temperate conditions of north India.

Anjan grass (*Cenchrus ciliaris*)

The genus *Cenchrus* is consisted of some 20 important species of annual and perennial grasses having an excellent forage values of which, *C. ciliaris* (Anjan grass or Kolukattai grass), *C. setigerus* (Black Kolukattai) and *C. glaucus* (Blue Buffel grass) are the most popular. It is also known with different name in different countries as buffel grass (Australia),and Afican foxtail (U.S. and Africa),

Among the three, the stem of Anjan grass (C. ciliaris) is of the thinnest stem as compared to the two others. The stem attends a height to about 150cm, bears drooping leaves with thin panicle making half circle curve. The tinny flowers mostly bear fertile seeds while the plant height of *C. cetigerus* is less than Anjan grass. It bears small broad leaf making a cup-shaped structure between leaf blade and leaf sheath. The panicles are also short and flowers are thinly placed. In *C. glaucus*, the leaves are pedecilated and panicles size is between the others two with awns (Photo 10).

Origin and History

It is an indigenous perennial grass and one of the popular pasture species in the arid and semi-arid region of Africa and India (Rajsthan, Punjab and Haryana states). Presently it is one of the major grassland species in N-W states of India. It was imported by the Australian where it is used as drought resistant grass and found an ideal grass for sheep.

Soil and Climate

Sandy to sandy soils with medium to high pH soils as well as saline soils of the arid climate is enough good for its production. Since, it is a draught resistant grass hence, usually fond fit in low rainfall areas. High rain fall regions with poor drainage system are not suitable for its survival.

Cultural Practices

Pasture is established during pre-monsoon after cleaning and ploughing the land to eradicate weeds and unpalatable bushes. It requires one year old seeds @ 5 kg/ha as the fresh seeds remained dormant. For quick and proper establishment basal application of 20 kgN + 10 kg P and topdressing of 20 kgN/ha after one month gives a good result In subsequent years too, application of 30-40 kg N/ha at the time of onset of monsoon should be done. As per growth 1-2 cutting or grazing is allowed at an interval of 6 weeks and 3-4 grazing in subsequent years.

Varieties

Some of the promising varieties have been developed by the different institutes for growing in their respective area.

Varieties	Characteristics
Marwar Anjan (CAZRI-75)	Developed for arid zone through clonal selection method from exotic line EC 14369 from Australia can be propagated by both seeds and rooted slips. It is erect type with indeterminate long panicle and dull spike, conical brown grains and remains green for longer period. Under rain fed conditions 9-10 t GF/ha and 4-5 t DM/ha can be taken
CO-1 (Neela Kokukattai)	Developed from clonal selection of FS-391 for south India that gives about 55 t GF/ha under rainfed conditions.
Bundel Anjan-1	Developed by intra population selection of IGFRI-S- 3108 is a semi-erect, thick stem, high tillering, large compact spike, purple nodes, droopy long-broad leaves. It is late maturing and resist both drought and frost. It is also very responsive to nutrient application and has potential yield of 35-40 t GF/ha.
Bundel Anjan-3 (IGFRI-727)	It is very suitable for arid and semi-arid central to western states which has high yield potential over other varieties.

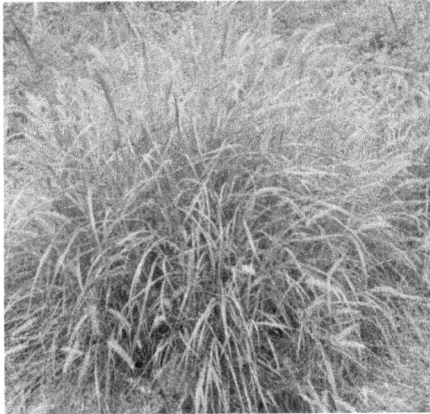

Photo 10. Anjan grass (*Cenchrus ciliaris*)

Package of Practices

Seeds production in this grass is quite sufficient therefore it is easy to establish through seeds in rangelands and pastures. Broadcast seeding of 25-30 kg seeds with fluff /ha in lightly prepared land is done as a surface seeding or just 1.5 cm below the soil surface. Under cultivated conditions, sowing of 5-7 kg seeds/ha at row - row distance of 30-40 cm and at 1-1.5 cm depth is done. It is also raised through planting of 40-50 days old seedlings at 40x20 cm. In some countries it is also grown as a component of ley-farming. In India, Bundel-1 and Marwar Anjan are grown under arid conditions of western India.

Under cut and carry system, first cutting can be taken after 80-90 days stage and subsequently at 6-7 weeks intervals. In low rainfall areas, 25-30 tonnes/ha of green herbage can be obtained with 27-30% dry matter content. The grass remains palatable even if, it is harvested at flowering. Therefore, it is also good for hay and silage making. The CP content also varies as such in younger plants it may be above 10% while in matured plant it may be as low as 5%. Some new genotypes through hybridization of *C. ciliaris* with *Pennisetum ciliare* have also been released which gives higher yield than their parents.

Rhodes grass (*Chloris gayana* Kunth.)

Genus *Chloris* Sw. (Posaceae) has about 100 species of annuals and perennials with semi-folded leaves and stolen type of root which gives birth to daughter plants. Inflorescence from 6-10 spreading rachis arising from one base are 5-8 cm long with thickly placed spikelets which changes to dull straw colour at ripening. Each seed is covered with about 2.5-3.0cm long lemma consisted of a pair of 2-5 cm awns (Photo 11).

Origin and History

The name Rhodes is referred to Cecil Rhodes of Cape Town, South Africa who popularized it as a forage crop. It was introduced to US and else where in early nineteenth century. In India, it is cultivated in Kernataka, Rajsthan and other low rainfall areas of neutral to alkaline and saline soils.

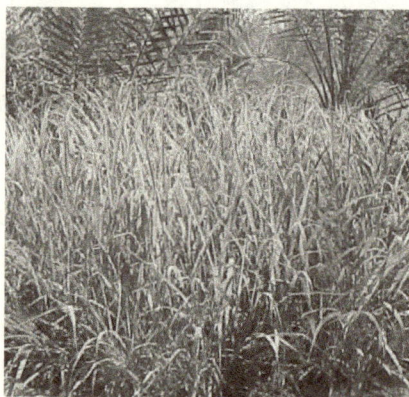

Photo 11. Rhodes grass (*Chloris gayana* Kunth.)

Soils and Climates

It gives good response in hot humid tropical climate but it can be produced in sub-tropical area as a drought tolerant grass. Heavy soils of high rain receiving areas are unfit for its growth. Sandy-loam soils of low rainfall regions and waste lands are ideal for its production. The soils with high pH as well as saline soils are better than low pH soils of high rainfall regions.

Package of Practices

Since, the seeds produced by this grass have excellent germination percentage hence, it is raised through seeds. Under natural conditions, 12-15 kg seed/ha is required for broadcasting. It is also propagated through rooted slips at row to row and plant to plant spacing of 50cm and 40cm, respectively .For a good stand of the grass, one weeding after 40-45 days of sowing or after 30 days of planting is done. If, the plant population of the sown grass is more, thinning and keeping optimum plants at 50x40 spacing helps in more tillers production and yield. Though, under grazing situation, manuring is seldom done but it gives a better yield under cut and carry system.

Cutting management and Yield

Crop is raised through vegetative method, first cutting can be taken after 6-8 weeks but it takes 10-12 weeks if, it is a sown grass. Under sub-tropical favourable conditions, 6-8 cuts while in coastal regions, it can give 10-12 cuts. This way, fresh yields of 40-50 tonns/ha in dry areas, 80-100 tonns/ha in sub-tropics and 140-180tonns/ha in tropics can be harvested. It is of average nutritive value with only 5-6%CP but a little adequate in calcium and phosphorus. It is better suited under grazing system than cuttings as it is also not good for silage but relatively good for hay.

Spear Grass (*Heteropogon contortus* Beauv.)

As it appears from the name itself that due to bearing of spear like very sharp awns attached with each seeds of the inflorescence, it is designated as spear grass. An indigenous semi-erect perennial and also distributed throughout the world forests. Now a day, it is found in almost all the forest areas of Northern India and also in some parts of South Indian states. It is usually managed under poor management conditions. Even it grows well on rocky soils on which its prostrate growth habit in early growth stage, make it possible as not to allow other species to come over. Plant height varies from 50-100 cm in different soil types (Photo 12).

Variety

Only a few progressive varieties of this grass have been developed. Among them Bundel Lampa Ghas-1 (IGHC 03-4) is developed for rangeland in drought prone areas of semi-arid, tropical and sub-tropical regions as a perennial by selecton from germplasm IG 95-284 collected from Datia, M.P.) It gives 25-30 t GF/ha and 8-10 t DM/ha.

Grazing/Cutting Management

This grass sustains well under frequent grazing conditions. Therefore, it is used as a range and pasture species rather as a cut forage. In some countries, it is used in short term pasture or leys in rotation with food or fibre crops. The livestock is allowed to graze at an interval of 6-7 weeks or as per growth of the plants. Green herbage generally contains 6-7% CP. Cutting or grazing is stopped at least 8-10 weeks earlier if the grass is to be harvested for seeds. Besides, *C. gayana; C. bournei* and *C. barbata* are also grown in some parts of the world.

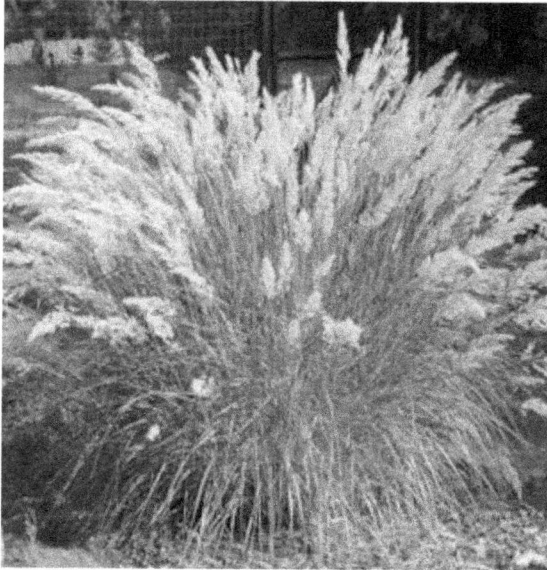

Photo 12. Spear Grass (*Heteropogon contortus*)

In addition to above medium to high yielding forage grasses, a few varieties of some of the other grass species have been developed. Though, having low yield potential but are the main component of natural and the largest grass cover of India *viz: Sehima-Dicanthium* cover. For example in Saem grass (*Semima nervosum*), Bundel Saem grass-1 (IGS 990) and in Marvel grass (*Dicanthium annulatum*), Marvel-7, Marvel-8, Marvel-93 and GMG-1 have been released for renovation of deterioted grasslands.

Chapter 5

Tropical Forage Legumes

Among the tropical forage legumes; some of them are grown as a cultivated forage crops or as a food and forage crops both. As a food crop, some are consumed by human being as pulses while others as green vegetables.

A. Cultivated

A very large number of tropical legumes are cultivated as forage as well as for both food and forage purposes. Among them, some of the most popular are:

1. Cowpea (*Vigna unguiculata*)
2. Ricebean (*Phaseolus calcaratus*)
3. Sunnhemp (*Crotalaria juncea*)
4. Forachis/Wild groundnut (*Arachis glaberata*)
5. Horsegram (*Dolichos biflorus*)
6. Field Bean (*Dolichos lablab*)
7. Soya bean (*Glycin max*)
8. French bean (*Phaseolus vulgaris*)
9. Broad bean (*Vicia faba*)
10. Yam bean (*Dolichos lablab* L.)
11. Greengram/Mung (*Phaseolus mungo*)

12. Blackgram (*P. calcaratus*)

13. Methi/ Fenugreek (*Trigonella foenum-graecum*)

14. Cluster beans (*Cyamopsis tetragonaloba*)

15. Pigeon pea/Red gram/Arhar (*Cajanus cajan*)

Cowpea (*Vigna unguiculata*)

The genus *Vigna*, generally a tropical trailing or twining herb, is consisted of over 60 species of forage and food crops. Besides its name as cowpea, it is also known as Lobia, Bodi and of course as a Cherry bean. Its vines may be of more than 1M long with tri-foliate broad leaves. Flower representing the typical characteristics of legume having 1 stander, 2 wings and 2 keels, looks like a butterfly with deep blue colour at the centre. It develops into a long pod. Though, forage types bear short pods but some vegetable types, pods are more glabrous as long as 50-60 cm. These pods contain kidney shaped seeds of several colours and sizes. (Photo 13)

Origin and History

Cowpea is being cultivated by the Romans, Espanis and Greeks since long as a food crop. Central Africa is considered to be the origin of this legume but India is also supposed to be the native place. Presently, it is one of the major pulse crop in Africa while, it is a major vegetable and forage crop in Indian continent.

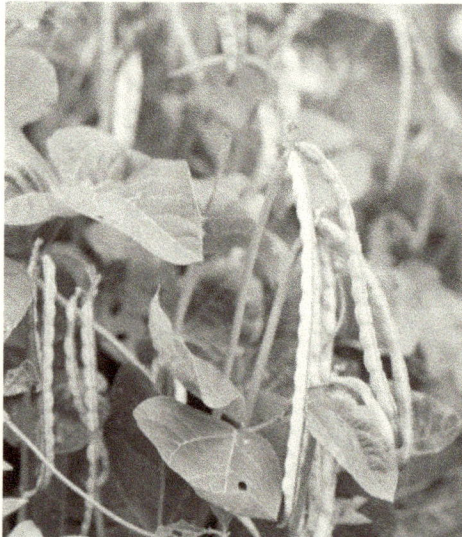

Photo 13. Cowpea (*Vigna unguiculata*)

Soils and Climate

Cowpea is most resistant to soil acidity among the cultivated tropical legumes. Therefore, it requires light sandy to loam soils of pH as low as 5.0 and as high as to neutral but low pH soils with high rainfall area is not suitable for its sowing since, the incidence of root rot at early growth stage has been reported. Hence, early sowings just before or just after the onset of monsoon is suggested. In these areas, performance of this crop is excellent as summer forage. Therefore, it is cultivated round the year except in chilly winter.

Package of Practices

The land is well prepared with 2-3 ploughings and planking. Basal addition of 8-10 tonnes compost/ha along with 20kgN/ha and 40kgP$_2$O$_5$/ha should be done. Though, line seeding at 30-40cm row to row and about 10cm seed to seed spacing is preferred but even broad casting also gives a good result. For forage production as pure stand, 60-70kg seed/ha is required but for seed production and as an intercrop, 25-35 kg seed/ha is sufficient. Cowpea is sown during early monsoon or as a summer crop in February-March in north India while, it is grown from October-January in south India. One hoeing and weeding at 3-4 weeks old crop should be done there after it does not required any cultural operation since the ground is fully covered with vines. This legume should be cut at the start of the first pod formation stage which, may vary from 60-70 days.

Varieties

Varieties	Characteristics
Kohinoor	Developed through single plant selection of variety from Iran (IL-68 786) is of 60-70 cm tall, stem and pods are green with bold-red seeds. It gives 40-45 t GF/ha and 4-5t DM/ha is more suitable for summer in north- west region.
Type-21	It is also developed through single plant selection from a local material gives 33 t GF/ha and 5 t DM/ha and suitable for all over the country.
Bundel Lobia-1 (IFC-8401)	Developed through single plant selection from IL-515 of 120-130 cm tall with 5-7 branches from basal and semi-tendrical. Rectangular to round seeds with gray dotting. It is grown in medium rainfall areas which gives 30-35 t GF and 4-5 t DM/ha at 65 days.

Contd...

Varieties	Characteristics
Bundel Lobia-2 (IFC-8503	It is a selection from IL-978 and good for north-west zone. Plant is 140-150 cm tall with erect to semi-erect 4-5 tendrical branches. Leave are broad of 15-20 cm long and seed is of fawn white with variable pinkish shade gives 30-35 t GF and 3.5-4.0 t DM/ha, contains 17% protein. Suitable for summer and low rainfall regions.
UPC-5286	Selected through a single plant, gives 35 t GF/ha and matures in 140-150 days
UPC-287	Single plant selection from germplasm line CK-72-287,takes 140 days for 50% flowering and produces 30-35 t GF/ha
UPC-4200	Developed through pure line selection from CK-76-4200 . Erect during early stage but changes to tendrical and climbing with profused branching with dark green foliage with broad globose leaflets. Light violet flower developes straw brown pods with kidney shaped medium size, testa colour black mottled seeds. It is grown in high humid areas and gives about 32 t GF/ha.
UPC-8705	Derived from a cross of N- 425 x H-288, takes 80-90 days for 50% flowering and 140-145 days for maturity.and produces 35-40 t GF/ha and more than 5 t DM/ha
UPC-9202	Produced from intervarietal cross between V-260 x UPC 9805-7-2-4 is a medium late variety (80-85 days), gives 35-40 t GF/ha, cultivated in central part of the country.
UPC-607	A cross of L-212 x Singapore-48-2-9 mature in 140-145 days is for growing in tropical and N-W India. It gives 35-40 t GF and 4.5-5.0 t DM/ha
UPC-618	Selection from the cross between UPC-8702 x IT-84E-124-2-5-1 is suited for all cowpea growing states of the country, matures in 140-150 days with medium yield (30 t GF/ha and 5 t DM/ha)
UPC-621	High yielding (50-55 t GF/ha and 6-8 t DM/ha) when cut at 50% flowering (85-90 days) variety for tarai region. Fit for intercropping with cereals has high digestibility and rich in protein (17%).
UPc-625	A dual purpose variety which lives green even after seed maturity. Seeds are creamy white with rough wrinkled testa is preferred as pulses. As a pulse crop it gives 6-8 q/ha grain and as a forage, cutting at 50% at 80-85 days it gives 35-40 t GF/ha and 5 t DM/ha is also compatible as an intercrop with cereals.
Fodder Cowpea-CO_8 (FCO-8)	A hybrid of CO-5 x N-331 is semi-spreading erect in early and creeping in late stages. It is grown round the year in south India as an inter crop with cereals. It is free from all types of diseases and leaf hopper. Plant attends 100-120 cm height and flowers at 60-70 days gives medium yield but high in protein (21%) and about 3% fat.
CL-367	Crossing of Cowpea 74 and strain No. 90 and bulked in F_6 generation evolved this variety is grown in irrigated area of Punjab as a short duration forage for about 25 t GF/ha.

Diseases and Pests Control

Crop sown during peak monsoon may be affected from root-rot disease just after emergence. Therefore, sowing should be completed during pre-monsoon or as late as just at the onset of monsoon. Seed treatment with 2% Bevistin may be effective to some extent.

Insects like; Hairy caterpillars at full growth period in the months of September- October is very common. It lays eggs on the dorsal sides of the leaves, as these developed in to caterpillars, start to eat the chlorophyll of the leaves which turn to white. These can be identified in the early morning as they live in group. The whole leaf is taken out and the small insects are killed.

The inflorescences are also affected by aphids, hence the crop may be harvested and fed or in extreme case, a very dilute solution of insecticide can be sprayed but the forage must be harvested after at least one week of spraying or after a spell of rain.

If, the crop is left for seed production, pods are damaged by weevils hence, one spraying of parathion or malathion @ 0.1-0.2% solution can done.

Cluster Beans/Guar (*Cyamopsis tetragonaloba* L. Taub.)

An erect annual of 1-1.5m height tropical legume with trifoliate pinnate leaves having dentate margin and stem bearing hairs is fond in Asia and Africa. It bears small purple flowers at the axils which, develops into a cluster of thick fleshy pods. These linear pods are consisted of compressed rounded 6-10 seeds which look like the seeds of cowpea. Green pods of some of the varieties are also used as table purposes. Guar is grown as a vegetable crop since long in Asia and is supposed to be indigenous to India.

Soils and Climate

It thrives well in light sandy to sandy loam soils of slightly acidic to neutral pH soils. Soils with high moisture retaining capacity are not suitable since relatively it is a drought resistant crop. High rainfall area of eastern India is not enough favourable for Guar growing while, arid region of north-west states are more ideal as such, it is one of the major pulse crop of Punjab, Haryana and Rajasthan where, it is also used as a green manure to raise the soil fertility. In some parts it is also cultivated as a forage crop as it needs less care in comparison to other monsoonal species.

Package of Practices

In North India sowing is done in February-March as summer irrigated crop but as a rainfed, its sowing is preferred in June-July. In South plateau the sowing is extended up to September-October. For forage purposes, Guar is usually seeded as broadcast with a seed rate from 25-30 kg/ha but for vegetable purposes 10-12 kg seed/ha are drilled at 40-45 cm apart and 6-8 cm from plant to plant. If the soil is poor in fertility, a basal dressing of 10-12 tonnes FYM/ha along with 20-25 kg N/ha and 40 kg P_2O_5/ha can give a good performance. Irrigation in summer crop should be given frequently as per requirement but in rainy season it seldom needs irrigation.

Varieties and Yield

Guara-80 is cultivated in Punjab and Haryana while, FS-277, HFG-119, HFG-156, IGFRI-212 and IGFRI-2395-2 are suitable for the whole India.

Small pods bearing types which, contains stiff hairs on the entire plant, are best suited for forage and green manure. Sirsa No. 1, No. 2 and Pusa Sadabahar are good types with more leaves and tall for multi-purposes including forage, green manure and to some extent also as a vegetable crop. As a forage crop, it is harvested at the first pod formation stage. Depending on the variation in start of reproductive phase, variation in cutting may be from 50-75 days after emergence. About 15-20 tonnes green herbage yield/ha with 18-20% dry matter and 16-18% CP can be harvested.

Rice Bean/Red Bean (*Vigna umbellate*, T / *Phaseolus calcaratus* R)

Rice bean (*Vigna umbellate* (Thumb.) / *Phaseolus calcaratus* belongs to family *Fabaceae* is a leguminous forage crop grown in rice growing hot humid climate of east and north India as an intercrop with maize. Like cowpea it thrives well in acid soil without liming. It is better than cowpea since it is neither damage by continuous heavy rain nor by Hairy catter pillar which is very common in Bengal, Bihar, Jharkhand and Odisha.

As intercrop with maize it requires 20 kg seed/ha in 2:1 pattern (Maize: Rice bean) during pre-monsoon as well as after early harvest of rice. Recently some varieties have been developed by BCKV, Kalyani (W B) and PAU Ludhiana (Punjab).

Varieties	Characteristics
Bidhan-1 (BC 15/K 1)	Developed after selection from a local landrace is 130-140 cm long tendrical, profused branching, light green stem with leaf ; stem ratio of almost 1:1. It bears yellow flower which develops in to 7-9 cm long pod containing 6-7 seeds/pod. It is drought resistant as well as tolerant to water logging, gives 35-40 t GF/ha, 20% CP and 2 t seed/ha.
Bidhan Rice Bean 2 (KRB 4)	It is also developed by local landrace selection for cultivation in N-E India. It is resistant to yellow mosaic virus and other pathogens which attack green gram and black gram. Attends 130-140 cm plant length which turns viny with a number of branches. Flowering starts in 110-120 days to produce about 40 t GF/ha and if left for seed production, it matures in 106-180 days and gives 2 t seed/ha.
RBL-1	It is the first variety released by PAU for growing in Punjab and Haryana.
RBL-6	It is a selection from the germ plasms collected from Nagaur (Rajasthan) is recommended for cultivation in whole of north India from Punjab to Bihar and Odisha. It is relatively short duration variety (105 days for forage and 120 days for seed). Plants are of spreading-viny, about 100 cm in length, light green leaves in lobed with fine hairs, and disease resistant, gives 15-20 t GF/ha.

B. Pasture/Range Legumes

Stylo (*Stylosanthes sps*)

Origin and History

Stylosanthes species is commonly known as Stylo belongs to the Tribe: *Aeshynomeneae*, Sub-tribe: *Stylosanthinae* Family: *Leguminosae* Sub-family: *Papiliosae* is first identified by Linnaeus (1753) as *Stylosanthes guianensis* and *Stylosanthes viscosa.* Latter on Aublet (1775) also identified *Trifolium gracilis* which was further known as *S. guianensis.* Swartz (1788) also recognized *S. guianensis* and *S. biflora* as a pasture legume. After one year he again evolved the other two *S. procumbens* and *S. elector* in 1789. Ferrina and Costa (1879) the two Brazilian scientists recognized 25 species including 9 new species while, on the other an Australian Mannetje (1967& 1977) also succeeded in evolving some new species of this genus.

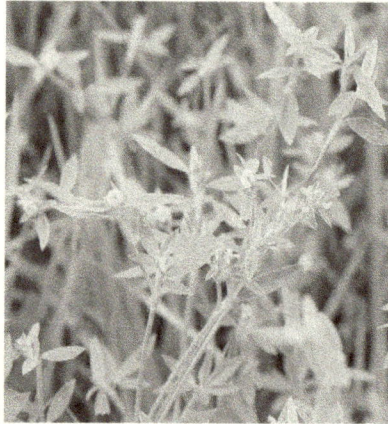

Photo 14. Stylo (*Stylosanthes guinensis*)

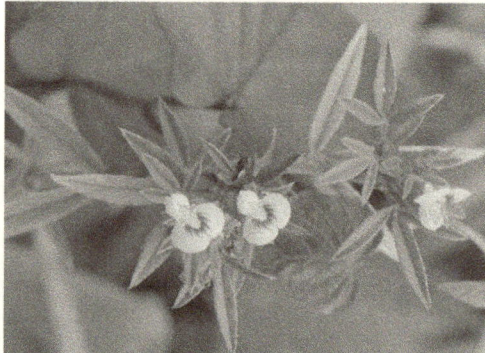

Photo 15. Stylo (*Stylosanthes hamata*)

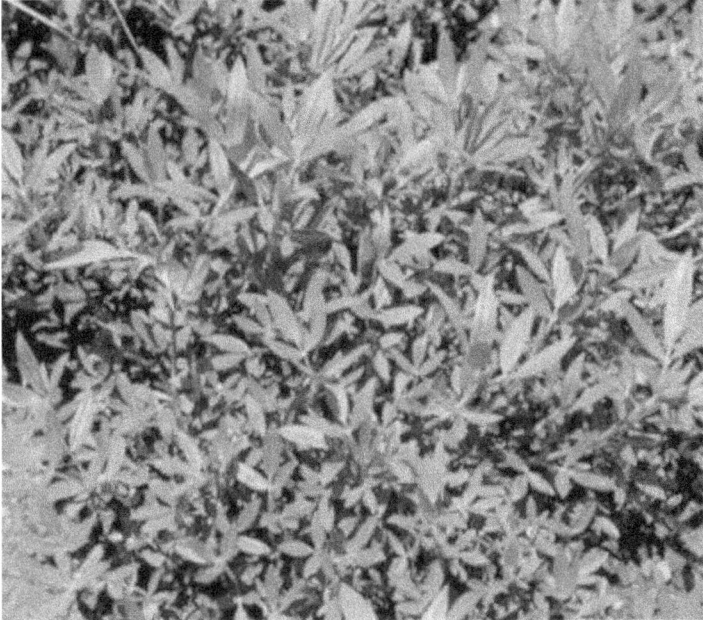

Photo 16. Stylo (*Stylosanthes humilis*)

Distribution and Introduction in India

The native place of majority of Stylo is in Latin American countries in general and Brazil in particular. A few of them are also having their home land in South Africa and North-Eastern Australia. Now a days it is widely grown as a leading pasture legume in Brazil, West-Indies, Australia, Hawaiian and Fizi islands as well as in sub-sahara region of East Africa. *Stylosanthes humilis* an annual and *S. gracilis* perennial drought resistant pasture legumes were first introduced at Ranchi (India) during 1954-55 from Australia. A large number of species *viz, S. scabra, S. hamata, S. fruticosa* including some new genotypes of *S. guianensis and* S. humilis were also imported from Australia by the Breeder at Ranchi in 1977. Latter on in 1992 two varieties of *S. guinensis viz*, Waynn and Amiga were also brought at Ranchi from Australia. Thus, Ranchi became the leading center for Stylo germplasms.

Plant Characteristics

"Stylos" in general are short day herbs of polyploidy series (x =10) with selfing as the breeding method. Plants vary in growth habit as per species, from erect woody stem to semi-erect or even prostrate. Stems as well as trifoliate leaves are covered with club-shaped hairs to reduce loss of water through transpiration. Some of them are also having gummy material on their leaves. The trifoliate leaves are mainly sessile with individual leaflets being long and flat in the middle and even narrow pointed at the tip in some other species (Photo 14, 15 and 16).

Table 5.1: Important species and cultivars with distinct characters

Sl.No.	Species	Cultivars	Characteristics
1	Townsville Stylo (*Stylosanthes humilis*)	Patterson, Lawson, Gordon and Kulumbara	Annual strain, thin-narrow leaves, seeds covered with hook like seed coat, prostrate with thin stems.
2	Brazilian Lucerne(*S. guianensis*)	Schofield, Graham, Cook, Endeavour, Amiga & Wynn	Prostrate to semi-erect perennial, trifoliate broad sessile leaves, late flowering seeds resemble like Lucerne seeds. Graham has thin stem as to Schofield.
3	River Hunter Lucerne/ Caribbean stylo(*S.hamata*)	Verano	Erect perennial early flowering, suitable for low as well as high pH soils.
4	Shrub Stylo(*S. scabra*)	Seca	Woody shrub, Broad-short leaves with sticky in touch, suitable for arid and semi-arid areas.
5	*S. fruticosa*	Q 41219	Erect with very small leaves low productive and less palatable
6	*S. viscosa*	Q 34904	–Do–
7	*S. mueronata*	--	–Do–

Characteristics for Growing in Acid Soils Conditions

Majority of the pasture lands are managed in acid soils of different countries throughout the world. These soils are toxic in iron and aluminium on one hand and deficient in organic matter, available essential nutrient elements such as N, P, Ca, B and Mo on the other. In addition, such soils are also in poor moisture retaining capacity but Stylo can sustain under these constraint conditions due to having following characteristics.

1. Deep and fine root systems facilitate it to extract moisture more efficiently under moisture stress conditions of the soils.

2. Since, leaves are consisted of less number of stomata and even

these are of sunken structure, reduce the loss of water through slowing down the transpiration rate.

3. Presence of hairs and gummy materials on the leaves and stems further reduces the rate of transpiration.

4. It is also very resistant to high light intensity and high summer temperature as high as 50°C but below 4°C, it suffers from cold injury.

5. It nodulates freely in low pH soils even in absence of Rhizobium culture.

6. It has very efficient built in mechanism for biological N-fixation and at the same time it has the capacity to self utilize about 90% of self fixed nitrogen. Thus, it is grown successfully in poor fertile soils of degraded rocky forests and even competes strongly with robust grasses like Hybrid Napier, Thin Napier, Guinea and several others.

7. According to one finding, its roots secret some alkaline chemicals which, changes the soils microclimate from acidic to neutral or even alkaline to increase the soil pH and hence, the unavailable form of nutrients like calcium and phosphorus change to available forms. Thus, it is grown in acid soils even without liming.

8. In another finding, its roots also secret some organic materials which combine with toxic elements to form complex ions. Since, these complex ions are bigger in size as compared to normal ions, their entry is restricted in to the xylem cells hence, and toxicity is eliminated.

9. The P requirement of this legume is the lowest (Available soil P<2.5 ppm) among most of the forage and grain legumes. This may be due to the fact that when the concentration of P in solution is increased, the upward flow of this nutrient in xylem vessels is restricted and hence, the P requirement is as such tends to the minimum level. Therefore, soils low in available-P is suitable for this legume.

Nutrients Requirement

Soils with > 2.5 ppm of available-P, does not give response to externally applied P. The concentration of calcium should be higher than 1.25 ppm. Since, it is resistant to aluminium toxicity hence, it can be grown even concentration of this element may be up to 75 ppm.

Though, the deficiencies of other nutrient elements are not very common however, increasing the levels of K, decreases the concentration of Ca, Mg and P at the exchangeable site.

Table 5.2: Nutrient Requirement Based on Plant Analysis

Nutrient	Critical level (%)	Optimum level (%)
P	0.16	0.19
K	1.00	0.19
Ca	1.50	5.00
Cu	0.05	0.05
S	0.12	0.12
Zn	0.34	0.34

The nutrients requirement of this pasture legume is very low as it thrives well on poor soils. Any how, for quick establishment, addition of 5-10 tonnes/ha of compost along with 20-25 kg N/ha+ 30-35 kg P_2O_5 +25-30 kg K_2O/ha as basal can be optimum.

Seed Treatment

It requires seed treatment before sowing due to hard seed coat which prevents easier germination. The seeds are first scarified and cleaned. These cleaned seeds are then put in concentrated sulphuric acid in one glass container for 10 minutes and thereafter it is washed 2-3 times in fresh water. Washed seeds are then dried in shade. If, the acid is not available, seeds can be soaked in fresh water for over night. Such treated seeds germinate in only 36-48 hours and gives better plant stand.

Seed rates and sowing

If the germination is 80-90 percent, 4-5 kg/ha of seeds are required for sole stand but as a mixture with grasses, 2-3 kg seeds/ha is enough. The seeds can be sown as broadcast from 1-1.5 cm below the soil surface for pasture purposes but for cut and carry system, it may be sown in alternate rows with grass at 40 cm spacing and not more than 2 cm below the ground surface. 1-2 ploughing, followed by one planking serves the purpose.

In degraded forest land and ravines, the aerial sowing is also done by the airplanes. The seeds are fixed in pellets of clay soil clods of 2-3 cm diameter and air dropped. This small quantity of soil facilitates germination on even rocky surface to establish the plants.

Grazing/Cutting Management

In the establishment year of sole legume or in association with grass in a pasture system, first grazing or cutting can be allowed in the month of September of June sown crop but if the stand of the legume is not satisfactory, the legume should be left for only seed production so that the self shattered seed can give an excellent cover in succeeding years. From the next year on ward depending on the growth, 2-3 grazing can be possible at an interval of 6 weeks. An annual pure stand of stylo can provide 25-30 tonnes green herbage/ha while perennial types can produce 35-40 tonnes green herbage/ha. These species contain about 20-25% of dry matter and fairly good amount of protein (14-16%). Among these species 'Schofield" variety of *S. guianensis* competes well with all the grasses in general and with the most robust thin Napier and Hybrid Napier in particular (Prasad, 1981).

Siratro (*Macroptilium atropurpureum*) and *M. lathyroides*

Atro the parent of Siratro, is a deep rooted trailing perennial with rooting habit at the nodes. This legume is pinnately-trifoliate, dark green with little hairy at the ventral side but silvery and very hairy at the dorsal side. Lateral leaflets, ovate, obtuse (4-6cm long). It has raceme inflorescence with10-30 cm long peduncle, 6-12 flowers crowded at the apex with deep purple having reddish twing near the base of the petals. Pods size varies from 7-9 cm long contains several seeds (4.0x2.5x2.0 mm) of brown to black in colour and of flattened shape (Photo 17).

Distribution: It is native to Mexico as well as to Matlopa in San Luis Potosi. It is also an natural vegetation in Central-South America. The present day Sitro is developed by E. M. Hutton (1970) in Queensland, Australia.

Soil and Climate: Sitro is a very important pasture legume of acid soils of low moisture retaining capacity. It prefers long day length of latitudes from 30°N to 28°S at temperature ranging from 26-30°C but it can survive even at 40°c It is very resistant to low soil pH (as low as 4.5) and also to drought condition as well as to high temperature (45°C). It nodulates freely in presence of native rhizobia. Seeds are scarified and treated in sulphuric acid (sp. Gr. 1.8) for 10 minutes and washed with fresh water before sowing for fast germination.

Cutting or grazing should be done by leaving 15 cm from ground level. It competes well with grasses. Digestibility is above 50% on dry matter basis with equally good in NFE (Nitrogen free extract).

Others qualities: Since, it is resistant to acid soils hence, Ca deficiency hardly occurs but it requires P and Mo. A normal plant may contain plant-P, 0.24%, K, 0.75% and Mo, 0.25 ppm. It also raises the soil-N by fixing 100-175 kg N/ha/yr.

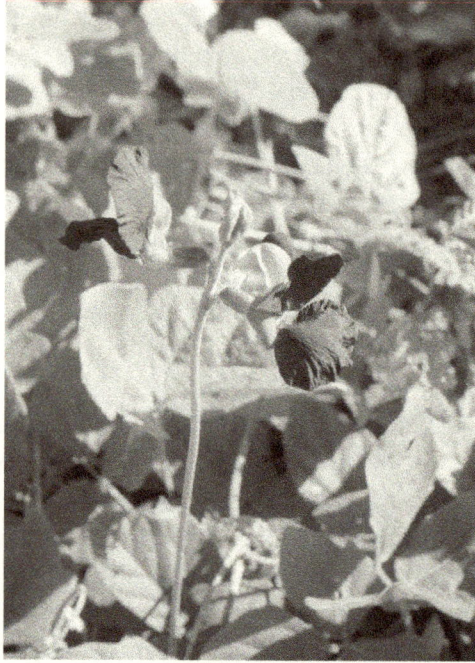

Photo 17. Siratro *(Macroptilium atropurpureum)*

Centro (*Centrosema* sps.)

Centrosema pubescens, Bench is known as Centro in Australia and elsewhere, in Argentina and Brazil as Jetirana and in Colombia as butterfly pea. Some of the other important species are: *C. brasilian (L.), C. pascorus, C. plumieri* and *C. virginianum* (L.).

It is a vigorous, trailing, twining and climbing perennial herb of 40-50 cm in length. The leaves are slightly hairy, trifoliate, dark green, ovate-elliptic and obtuse with 4.0x3.5 cm size. The dorsal part is hairy. Long stipples bear large showy flower in axillary raceme. Each flower has 2 striate branchcteoles. Pods are linear 7.5x15.0 cm long and flat thick twisted with 20 seeds of 4-5x3x4cm size having brownish black dark blotches (Photo 18).

Distribution: It is well distributed in South America from where it was introduced to Indonesia, India and other tropical countries lying between both 23°N and S latitudes at 600-900 elevation.

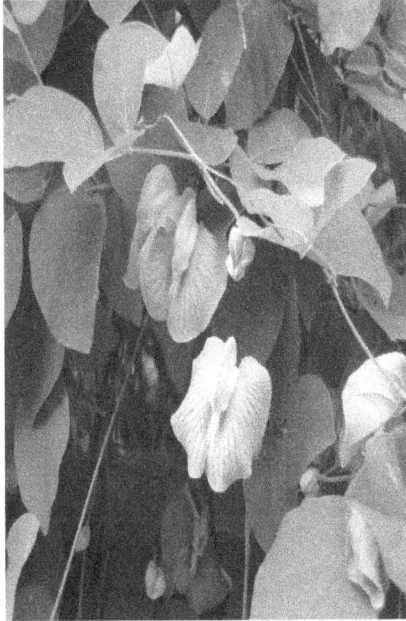

Photo 18. Centro (*Centrosema sps.*)

Soils and Climate

Temperatures of 26-32°C with rainfall from 120-140 cm is ideal conditions for its optimum growth. In high rainfall area, the soil water retaining capacity should be low since, it is one of the drought resistant pasture legume. It can be grown in low to high pH soils even in absence of external rhizobium culture.

Seed Treatment

To facilitate easier germination, scarification and dipping of seeds for 7 minutes in 24-36N-H_2SO_4 followed by washing in fresh water is required. Seeds can also be soaked for over night in water or in hot water of 75-80°C for 15 minutes.

Yield and Nutritive Values

Cutting or grazing should be only allowed from second year. As a sole crop about 100-125 q green herbage/ha can be obtained but it is better to grow with perennial grasses. If it is left for seeds production, it may give 225-275 kg seeds/ha.

A normal plant with optimum productivity contains 1.4% Ca, 0.16% P, 1.35-1.90% K and 16.5 ppm Cu.

Kudzu vine (*Puraria thunbergia*)/

Tropical Kudzu (*P. phaseoloides*)

Over a dozen species of *Puraria* genus is available in East Asia, East Africa and East Indies and introduced in India during 1927 as a forage and soil binding crop. These are relatively rough fast growing trailing perennials spread through rooting at the nodes and attend the length of 8-10 M. These vines tangle to each other and make harvesting difficult. The tri-foliate, stipulated large leaves are coarse in touch since, these contain a very high per cent of iron as the legumes are very resistant to low pH soils having toxic levels of both iron as well as aluminium. The long axillary racemes bear purple to light blue flowers which develop into thin long pods of long hilum containing orbicular seeds (Photo 19).

Package of Practices

Kudzu as a tropical legume favours hot-humid climate of high rainfall area but a soil of good drainage system. Low pH red soils of light texture with low moisture retaining capacity are suitable for this spreading legume. It is propagated from seeds as a broadcast system or inter cropped with perennial grasses.

About 8-10 kg seeds/ha is needed for pure seeding but with grasses 4-5 kg seeds/ha is sufficient. Its germination and growth are also very quick. If, it is harvested in younger age, it is good forage but it is rough just after flowering and even more at pods setting stages.

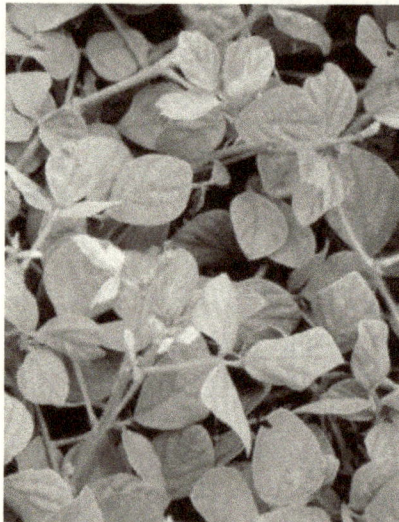

Photo 19. Kudzu vine (*Puraria thunbergia*)

Some of the other low yielding tropical legumes *viz*: Sem (*Lablab purpureus*) an African origin is also grown in some parts of which two forage types GACD-1 and Bundel Sem-1 (JLP-4) are developed for neutral to high pH soils.

Chapter 6

Temperate Forage Crops

Cereal Forage Crops

There is a very limited number of temperate cereals forage crops are available of which oat is the major one, cultivated under temperate conditions of Europe and sub-temperate conditions of India and elsewhere to the extent of 23° towards both sides of equator during winter season.

Oats (*Avena sativa* Linn.)

Origin and Distribution

Since, oats is a temperate forage crops and widely cultivated in temperate regions of the world, probably its origin appeared to be Europe or Western Asia. The cultivated oats is supposed to be a selection of either from Red oats (42) *Avena byzantica* or Wild oats (42) *Avena sterlis* (Kipps,1970). This genus has self pollinated of about 72 species distributed through out the world. It is cultivated in UK, USA, Russia, Canada Poland, France, Germany, North India and high lands of Eastern African countries. In India it covers about 500 000 ha land of which maximum area is occupied by UP(34%) followed by Punjab (20%), Bihar (16%), Haryana (9%) and Madhya Pradesh (6%).

Plant Characteristics

An erect to spreading annual plant of 1.25 to 1.75m tall, fibrous and hollow stem with solitary, alternate leaves of 25 to 1.5m long and 2-4cm broad sessile . Internodes are covered with leaf sheath. It bears equilateral or unilateral inflorescence with main axis and lateral branches end in a single apical spikelet. The panicle with one axis bears from 4-6 whorls of branches and the grain is covered with lemma and palea. Long spidle shaped seed are covered with puffs at the apex. The plant before flowering can be distinguished with wheat and barley as the barley plant has well developed over lapping auricle while in wheat, it is partially developed but in oats, it is completely absent (Photo 20).

Soils and Climate

It performs well in slightly acidic to medium alkaline and saline soils of sandy to sandy loam texture with good drainage conditions. Soils with medium to high infertility with irrigation are the most favourable for this forage crop. Its cultivation is extended from temperate to sub-tropical conditions. It requires an average maximum temperature of 25°C and average minimum temperature of 15°C for germination. For tillering phage, it requires low temperature of 20°C average maximum and 10°C of average minimum coincided with the shortest day length. For reproductive phase, a relatively higher temperature of 30°c and long day length is required. Any temperature above 35°C is injurious for grain production.

Package of Practices

One ploughing with soil turning plough followed by 2-3 with cultivators and planking are done to prepare a fine tilth. Generally line sowing at row to row spacing of 25 cm and in 4-5 cm furrow depth with 100-125 kg seeds/ha is done. The seed rate can be increased in late seeding. Under North Indian conditions, 1st to 15th November sowing gives the highest green forage yield (Rai *et al.*, 1976) however, for continuous supply of forage, it can be sown from mid-October to mid-December. Under Agroclimatic conditions of Ranchi, mid-November sowing and cutting at 80 days after sowing produced the maximum herbage however, for two cuttings, first cut at 50-55 days of seeding and second at 50% flowering may be taken (Prasad *et al.*, 1988)

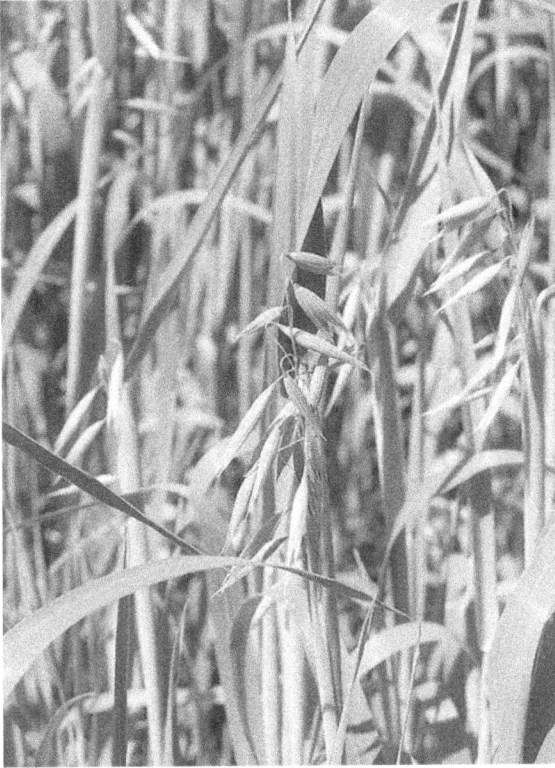

Photo 20. Oats (*Avena sativa*)

Application of 10-12 tonnes FYM/ha with 80kg N, 40 kg P_2O_5/ha and 30 kg K_2O/ha gives a good yield of both green herbage and grain. Level of N can be splitted as 1/3 rd as basal and half of the rest at crown root initiation stage and last after first cutting at 55-60 days of sowing or if, it is for seed production, the last dose can be top-dressed at flag leaf stage where as full dose of P and K are also applied at sowing. After sowing, one hoeing and weeding at 20-25 days followed by next after first cut should be done. Bhagat *et al.* (1985) suggested to apply 90kgN/ha as basal and 30kgN/ha as foliar spray at 60-70 days after sowing to harvest the maximum yield of green (60 tones/ha) and dry matter (12.4 tones/ha).

Application of 20kg $ZnSO_4$/ha in slightly alkaline soils (pH 7.1) containing 0.8 ppm available Zn along with 75kgN through urea and 25kgN through FYM was suggested to grow oats in molisol(Joshi *et al.*,2007) while Kumar and Ramawat (2006) advocated application of 40kgS/ha in sulphure deficient (8.0ppm) soils of temperate region of north India.

Irrigation

It gives higher yield under irrigated conditions. Alike wheat, these irrigations should be applied at the different critical growth stages which are;

(a) At emergence stage or just 2-3 days after sowing if, the soil has insufficient moisture for germination,

(b) At tillering or after 21-25 days after sowing,

(c) Stem elongation or boot stage,

(d) Flag leaf initiation or at last leaf stage and

(e) Dough or milking to grain feeling stages

The number of irrigations will also depend on soil types and their moisture retaining capacity. As such heavy soils, only 3 irrigations can serve the purpose while light textured soils with low moisture retaining capacity may require more than 5 irrigations. In some of the countries, it is cultivated fully as a rainfed crop where, the rainfall usually occurs from 700-800 mm.

Cutting Management

Generally, 2 cuttings are taken, of which 1st at 50-60 days after sowing when the crop attends 40-50 cm plant height, followed by second at 50% flowering stage. In some of the single cut varieties, only one cut at 50% flowering is taken. Bourah and Mathur (1979) suggested cutting of oats for forage at late milk stage for single cut system while at boot and late milk stages for 2 cut system. For seed production, either no cutting is taken or the crop is left for seeds after the 1st cut. Under 2 cut system, 30-35 tonnes green forage/ha and under single cut about 40-50 tonnes green forage/ha can be harvested. In 2 cuts system, 16-18% dry matter and 10-12% CP while in single cut 20-22% dry matter and 8-9% CP can be obtained. As a fully grain crop 2.5-3.0 tonnes grain/ha while grain after one cut as forage may give 1.2-15 tonnes grains/ha.

Serum of oats grains decreases the cholesterol level of blood, may be due to β-glucans. Furfural extracted from oats hulls, is used as a solvent for refining mineral and vegetable oils. It also contains high amino-acids but it is low in lysine content.

Varieties

More than two dozens of varieties have released by different Institutes of the country since 1974 and onwards. Among them about one and half dozen are the most promising.

Varieties	Characteristics
HFO-114 (Haryana Javi-114)	Developed by pure line selection is an early sown variety with good tillering capacity, tall, synchronized flowering with bold seeds. It is recommended for growing in all the oats growing states which produces 50-55 t GF/ha and 13 t DM/ha in two cuts as well as 2 t seed/ha.
Algerian	It is 100-125 cm tall, decumbent, 2-3 stout culms, slow early growth, pubescence on leafsheath, ligule of light green colour, 12-15 cm long and 10-12 cm thick panickle with straight rachis. It gives 40-45 t GF/ha
FOS-1/29	Prostrate plant with profuse tillering, narrow leaves and slow early growth. Grown as rainfed in N-W India. It gives 40-45 t GF/ha.
Kent	It is an introduction from USA in 1975 and still one of the widely grown varieties in entire country. Erect medium late type, 75-80 cm tall with long droopy leaves is resistant to lodging and diseases. It produces 45-50 t GF/ha if sown in first half November.
OS-6	Evolved from the crossing of HFO 10 x HFO 55 P2 has early vigour, tall, broad leaves of light green colour and medium bold seeds. Flag leaf remains erect at emergence of panicle, tolerant to diseases, performs well under sub-temperate and sub- tropical regions giving 54 t/ha green fodder in a single cut.
OS-7	The variety is a progeny of the cross between HFO 10 x HFO 55 P2. The variety has early vigour, tall, broad leaves of light green colour, medium bold seeds. Flag leaf remains erect at emergence of panicle, tolerant to diseases. The variety performs well under sub-temperate and sub- tropical regions of the country and also suitable for two cuts under irrigated areas of Haryana. The variety has early vigour tall, broad light green colour leaves and medium bold seeds. The green fodder yield is 69 t/ha and dry fodder is 12.5 t/ha.
Bundel Jal-822	A multi- cut variety developed from a cross between IGO-4268 X Indio-6–5-1 following intervarietal hybridization and pedigree method of selection for cultivation in central zone of the country. The variety has erect growth habit and glabrous nodes, takes 95-100 days for flowering and matures in 125-130 days and gives 50 t GF/ha and 12 t DM/ha.
UPO-212	The variety was developed by intervarietal hybridization (VS- 1492 X Kent) followed by pedigree breeding and selection for cultivation in the north and central India under multi-cut system has light green stem with 8-10 tillers, thin and variable awns. It flowers in 140-150 days. The average green fodder yield is 60 t /ha..

Contd....

Varieties	Characteristics
OL -125	The variety was developed by intervarietal hybridization using Appler and IPC – 163 followed by pedigree breeding and selection for cultivation in north- west and country. This is suitable for single cut/ multi cut and yields 58 t/ha green fodder.
Haryana Javi-8 (HJ-8)	The variety was developed from OS- 7 X S-3021 P for Haryana. It has fast growth better regeneration and suitable for two cuts. The flag leaf of the variety remains erect at the time of panicle emergence and panicle is straight and open. The variety provides 65 t/ha green fodder.
Sabzaar (SKO-7)	The variety has been notified for cultivation in temperate areas of Kashmir at high altitude regions of Jammu. The variety is of profused tillering, leafy and suitable for dual purpose. It produces 35-40 t/ha of green fodder.
Bundel Jai- 851	The variety was developed through selection from exotic Japanese germplasm "Hidgo Karyokuro". This is a multicut variety having fast regeneration and high protein content. It can give up to 4 cuts. Takes 110-115 days for flowering and 140-145 days for seed setting. It has prostrate growth habit but becomes erect after tillering. It gives 47 t/ha. of green and 8t/ha of dry fodder. The seed yield is 1.2 t/ha and crude protein yield 0.99 t/ha. The variety possesses desirable traits such as high regeneration potential, multicut nature (up to 4 cuts), high leafiness, high tillering and high crude protein.
Bundel Jai 992 (JHO 99-2)	A single cut variety developed through intervarietal hybridization followed by pedigree method of selection is of medium plant height, flowers in 100-105 days and matures in 140-145 days for N-W zone. It produces 50 t GF/ha and 10 t DM/ha with high protein (10.7%).
Bundel Jai 2004 (JHO 2000-4)	Developed through interspecific hybridization (*A. sativa*-JHO 851 x *A. m*acroccana- 16/30) followed by induced polyploidy and pedigree method of selection is a single cut variety for all the oats growing states. It gives 50 t GF/ha and 10 t DM/ha with 11% protein. It is also tolerant to all the fungal diseases.
Bundel Jai 99-1 (JHO 99-1)	Product of hybridization between OS7 x IGO320-1139-19 followed by prdigree method of hybridization for hilly region as a single cut. is resistant to grasshoppers, aphids and blight.in single cut at 120-125 days it gives 30 t GF/ha and 7 t DM/ha with 10% CP.
Bunder Jai 2001-3 (JHO 2001-3)	Developed from three way intervarietal hybridization (UPO 94 x IGO 320) x Akiyutaka followed by pedigree method of selection. It is a single cut prostrate but erect at later stage of growth suitable for N-W and southern zones of the country, gives 50 t GF/ha, 20 t DM/ha and contains 9% CP.
Harita (RO-19)	It is a selection from base population of Kent for Maharastra, gives on an average 50 t GF/ha with 9.5% CP.

Nitrate Toxicity

Nitrate toxicity in oats occurs, when herbage grown under very high level of nitrogenous fertilizer and if, the same herbage is prepared for hay and it is any how moist, the nitrate toxicity is developed. The NO_3^- under moist conditions in presence of micro-organisms changed to NO_2^- which is absorbed by ferrous form of iron found in hemoglobin is changed to met hemoglobin as the ferrous form of iron changed to ferric form and is precipitated or say, the blood is broken down. Since, met hemoglobin is a non-oxygen carrier hence the blood is devoid of oxygen, causes distress and death of the animal. If, even 30-40% of blood is changed into met hemoglobin, it results in 80-90% casualty.

Pests and diseases

In acid soils, the seeds are damaged by termites which can be controlled by application of 10% Aldrin dust @ 20-25 kg/ha at the time of sowing. It can be mixed with seeds itself.

Soil born disease like root rot caused by either *Helminthosporium vicoriae, Colletotricum graminicola or Fusarium graminarium* and other species in which discoloration of roots and bases of culms, yellowing of foliage and death of adult plants are common in alkaline soils. This can be controlled by summer fallows and timely sowing and use of resistant cultivars.

Stem rust caused by *Puccinia graminis* is the other disease in which pustules are formed on the leaves and stems with brick-red colour. It is more serious under moist conditions. Spraying of Dithane Z-78 @ 2 gm/litre of water or Bevistin @ 2.5 gm/litre can control the rust.

Loose smut caused by *Ustilago avenae* at the time of emergence of panicle is very common in some of the varieties. It changes the panicles in to full of black spores and finally the panicles look like skeletons. Since, it is a seed born disease hence treatment of the seeds before sowing with organo-mercuric fungicides, either Arasan, Spergon, Agrosan G N, Thirum or Bevistin@ 2.0-2.5 gm/kg of seeds can control this disease.

Temperate Grasses

Kikuyu grass (*Pennisetum clandestinum* Hochst. Ex Chiov)

The name is given after the Kikuya tribal of Kenya, east of the Aberdare Mountains. It is a natural habitat of the high lands (2,000 - 3,500m) of East and Central Africa including Ethiopia, Kenya, Uganda and Zaire. Kikuyu is further introduced to Costa Rica, Colombia, Hawaii, Australia (NSW) and Southern Africa from Zaire and Kenya. In India, it is introduced in hilly region of Neelgree high land from Kenya.

Plant Characteristic

This grass is a prostrate perennial to 40-50cm height, spreading through rhizomes and stolons due to rooting at the nodes. Leaves are 5-11 cm long and 0.5-0.7 cm in width with hairs. Ligules are with a ring of hairs with yellow coloured collar. It bears small flower in the upper most leaf-sheath. The spikelets are bi-sexual but functionally unisexual which bears 2mm long dark brown seeds.

Soil and Climate

Deep red soil of highlands with good drainage (latosolic soils) facility is required for its average performance but for higher productivity fertile alluvial soils is more ideal. It is also tolerant to salinity. High lands falling within both 27°N and S latitudes and up to 3500m altitude of 1000-1600 mm rainfall/year with mean 1270 ± 630 mm is congenial. Since, it is a deep rooted (5.5 m) grass hence, it tolerates drought and even can survive in 10 days of flooding. In high land, it grows well in spring, summer and autumn seasons as there is not much variations in temperature. It requires 20-30°C temperature for germination, and 16-21°C for optimum growth

Nutrient Requirement

Though, hardly any fertilizer is added in this grass, however it gives good response to nitrogen up to 120-150 kg N/ha/yr. About 17-24 kg DM/ha/kg N can be harvested. Mixed or intercropping with White clover (*T. repens*), reduces the N requirement. Least response to P was recorded but it needs K and S on heavy grazing conditions.

Methods of Sowing: After preparation of a fine tilth, hand planting of stem and root cuttings with 2-3 nodes at 1.0m spacing is done. In case of seed sowing, it is sown at 5mm soil depth.

Grazing/cutting Management

Light grazing is done to protect the stolons. Depending on the growth, cutting can be taken at 2-3 weeks intervals. Application of 22.4 kg N/ha/cut gives about 170-180q GFY/ha. It is an average in tolerance to fire.

Yield and Chemical Composition: In Australia (NSW), 30 tonnes of green herbage/ha/yr at 120kg N/ha was harvested. 25 kg seeds/ha from new crop and 500 kg seeds/ha from old stand were also harvested. Leaves contain 12%CP with 60-70 % digestibility. The P, K, Ca and Mg contents were also adequate.

Varieties

There are some good cultivars grown in African high lands. Among these, **Rongai** is of broad leaves where as **Kabete** is of medium type and **Molo** is of narrow leaves type. There are two others varieties, one is **Whittet** of taller, coarse, broad leaves and vigorous plant type where as, **Breakwell** is consisted of dense tillers, more prostrate with narrow leaves, thin stem and shorter internodes of which 15-20 seeds are male sterile and rest fully female fertile. All are relatively resistant to pest and diseases.

Animal Production

Kikuya based pasture + 336 kg N/ha/yr with 5 cows/ha produced 447 kg and 361 kg butter fat/ha in 2 lactations (Kaiser & Colman, 1969, NSW). It has also an economical value to check soil loss from erosion in high lands of tropical and sub-tropical countries.

Chapter 7

Temperate Forage Legumes

Clovers (*Trifolium species*)

The genus *Trifolium* (L) belongs to family Leguminoseae, sub-family Papilionaceae is consisted of about 300 sub-tropical to temperate species of which clovers, berseem, trefoils and shamrock are some of the important legumes used as forages. It is an erect to semi-erect annuals and a few perennials of 60-90 cm long hollow stems, trifoliate sessile leaves with entire or denticulate margin, small flowers on crown or head of white to yellow or purple red in colours, containing one to two oval shaped brown seeds within the calyx (Photo 21).

Clovers are the most valuable forage crop in temperate countries like, UK, US, Australia, New Zealand and high lands of African countries. In India, berseem (*T. alexandrinum*) and shaftal (*T. resupinatum*) are the two species widely grown as forage crops under irrigated conditions.

Some of the important species grown as a forage and pasture

S. No.	Common Name	Scientific Name	Origin
1.	Egyptian Clover/ Berseem	Trifolium alexandrinum	Egypt
2.	Shaftal/Persian Clover	T. resupinatum	Persia
3.	White Clover/Ladino Clover	T. repense	Europe
4.	Red Clover	T. pretense	W. Asia
5.	Crimson Clover	T. incarnatum	Europe

Contd...

Contd...,

S. No.	Common Name	Scientific Name	Origin
6.	Subterranean Clover	*T. subterranium*	Asia Minor
7.	Strawberry Clover	*T. fragiferum*	Australia
8.	Semipilosum	*T. semipilosum*	E. Africa
9.	Burchell	*T. burchellinum*	E. Africa
10.	Alsike Clover	*T. hybridum*	Sweden

Berseem/ Egyptian clover (*T. alexandrinum*)

Origin and Distribution

It is indicative from the name itself that it was originated from Egypt where, it is the principal forage crop of the country including Persia, Syria and other neighbouring countries. It also became the main winter forage crop of North, West and North-Eastern India since its introduction in 1916. It is usually grown in rice soils either as *paira* crop or just after the harvest of early maturing rice varieties from mid-October to November.

Soils and Climate

It is grown in sandy-loam to clay-loam soils with high in organic matter and from slightly acidic to alkaline soils as it is also used to reclaim such soils. It requires relatively high temperature (20-28°C) for germination and low temperature (10-15°C) followed by short to neutral day for vegetative growth and further high temperature (30-35°C) and neutral day length for flowering and seed formation. It is difficult to grow at high altitude above 1500 m having temperature nearer to frost.

Package of Practices

Seed treatment: It needs two types of seed treatments of which the first to separate the chicory and other weed seeds. The cleaned seeds are put into the 10% common salt solution in water. Since, the seed of berseem is heavier than weed seeds it deposited at the bottom of the pot and thus the floating chicory and other weed seeds are taken out and berseem seeds are washed in fresh water and dried in shade.

Secondly, if the crop is to be grown in the plots where it has not been grown earlier, it is preferred to inoculate the seeds with *Rhizobium* culture. Seeds are treated with *Rhizobium trifolii* bacteria. About 500 g of culture is mixed with per 10 kg of above salt treated seeds. Mixing of 500g of molasses or raw sugar with culture facilitates rapid growth of bacteria however, particularly in acid soils, it attracts the termites hence application of 20-25 kg of Aldrin dust is also required. After the treatment it should be dried again in shade but strictly not in the sun light since, it will kill the bacteria. If, the Rhizobium culture is not available, the soils of last year berseem cultivated plots can be used. Few kg of such soils are dried, powdered and mixing with the seeds serves the purpose. If the soils are high in organic matter, the plant roots are efficient to multiply the bacteria even it is devoid of external bacteria since some population of bacteria are usually present in the soil rhizosphere.

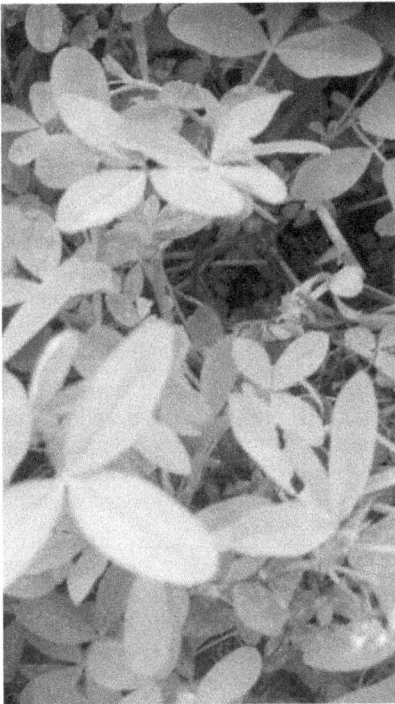

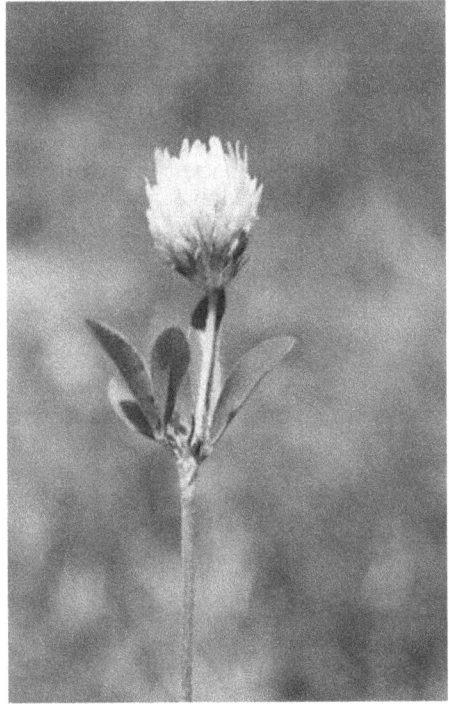

Photo 21. Berseem/ Egyptian Clover (*T. alexandrinum*)

Methods of Sowing

Berseem is sown with three methods. Seeds are sown in standing rice crop as a *Paira* crop before 2 to 3 weeks harvesting of the rice crop but if, the rice crop stand is very good, the germination of berseem will be poor which can be adjusted with high seed rate of the forage legume.

In early harvested rice crop, the sowing is preferred in puddle soils. The soil is puddle and planked and water is drained before broad casting the seeds. In medium land, dry sowing followed by light irrigation is preferred. The plot is ploughed to make fine tilth and seeds are either sown in rows or broadcast after light planking. Basal application of 20-25 tonnes FYM/ha along with 20-25 kg N/ha and 40-50 kg P_2O_5/ha gives more number of cuttings and yield. If the soil is deficient in Boron (<0.5ppm) and Molybdenum (<0.02 ppm), application of Borax (2-4 kg/ha) and Sodium or Ammonium –molybdate (0.25-0.50 kg/ha) can be done at sowing time by mixing the chemicals with fine sands or soils. Prasad *et al.* (1985) recommended application of 40kgN/ha with 36kgP/ha along with 5 tons compost/ha in 'Mescavi' besseem to harvest 75 tonnes of green and 11tons of dry herbages.

Varieties	Characteristics
Pusa Giant	An auto-tetraploid variety developed from the diploid variety C-10 has dark green broader and thicker leaves than those of diploid. Tetra and penta foliate leaves has also bigger flower than diploids and double inflorescence/plant. It gives 10-15% more forage than Mescavi and more winter and frost resistant.
Mescavi	Introduced from Egypt and then selected in India is fit for growing in entire country. It is shrubby and erect (45-75 cm) with profused branching at the crown, rounded at the tip, bright green and slightly hairy, Flower heads are white and round to give small seeds (2.7 g/ 1 000 seeds) yellow to brown colour. In 4-6 cuts, 65-70 t GF/ha is taken
Berseem Ludhiana	The variety has been bred through selection from Mescavi. It is adapted to Punjab situation. It is quick growing diploid variety that produces more branches than Mescavi. Its first cutting is ready about a week earlier than that of Mescavi and continues to supply green forage up to the end of May about 2 weeds late than Mescav yielding 80-110 t GF/ha
Jawahar Berseem-1	The variety has been developed from single plant selection from Chindwara followed by pedigree method of selection. It is recommended for cultivation in all berseem growing areas of the country especially central and north western zones. The average plant height is 47 cm; average number of branches is 5.2 and leaf: stem ratio is 1.61. Fully developed inflorescence is cylindrical and elongated in shape. Its productivity is 70-75 t/ GFha. This is a diploid variety of slow growth in cold temperatures and fast in rising temperatures at the end of winter season.
Wardan	The variety has been evolved through selection from the large genetically diverse polyploidy material. The plant habit is erect, white flower. 50% flowering at 150-165 days, and maturity in 175-190 days, Head colour is brown which possess 80-90 pale yellow coloured seeds. It provides green fodder yield 70-75 t/ha and dry 12-15 t/ha. A diploid type with slow growth in cold temperatures and fast in rising temperatures at the end of winter season.

Contd...

Contd...

UPB-10	The variety has been developed by developing composite of 5 lines followed by selection. It has prolific crown branching with succulent thick stem. The basal shoots and side branches develop freely after cutting, It matures in 200-210 days. The seed size is medium bold and colour is bright yellow and green forage yield is 70-75 t/ha.
Bundel Berseem-2 (JHB-146)	The variety has been bred through mass selection from indigenous material no. 25776 followed by pedigree selection. This variety flowers in 150-160 days and matures in 180-190 days. The plant height ranges from 55-65 cm under optimal cutting regime. It has dark green leaves. The crop is fairly tolerant to acidic conditions and is fertilizer responsive. The green forage yield is 90-100 t/ha. It is released for cultivation in central zone.
Bundel Berseem-3	The variety has beern bred through colchiploidy followed by recurrent single plant selection and then mass selection of the parent material JHB- 83-3, 1-90-P3-g-bl-hs-sb. The plants are erect with white flowers achieving 50% flowering in 155-170 days and maturity in 175-185 days. The variety is moderately resistant to stem rot and root rot diseases and has mean green fodder yield of 50-55 t/ha and dry fodder 8-10 t/ha. It is released for north east zone.
BL-22	Developed from irradiated material of Mescavi followed by pedigree selection. It gives 70 t GF/ha and supply forage at the end of June in temperate north-west zone.
JB-5	The variety has been developed through recurrent selection from the colchicine treated seed material has been recommended for cultivation in irrigated areas. It matures in 185-195 days and the average green fodder yield in 48 t/ha.
Hisar Berseem-1 (HFB-600)	The variety has been developed through selection from germplasm lines no. 6(307011, 11-OP). It is different from Mescavi in form of head shape and has medium maturity of 205-210 days. It yields 75t/ha green fodder and suitable for late sowing in hilly areas of the country.
BL-180	The variety has been developed by irradiation of BL 10 followed by selection. The variety has been released for cultivation in north region. The variety matures in 260-265 days and the average yield under normal conditions is 60-65 t/ha It is capable of supplying green fodder late in the season.

For sowing in standing rice crop, about 30kg seed/ha is used while for puddle and dry sowings 20-25 kg seed/ha is sufficient, if the germination may be above 90%. In mixed and intercropping, the seed rate is reduced to half and adjusted on row ratio, respectively. In mixed stand, some times, full seed rates of both the component species are applied.

Cutting Management and Yields

Berseem requires one nipping at the 5-6 leaf stage, in which upper 2-3 leaves along with bud are removed. This facilitates faster re-growth due to activation of the growth enzymes. There after the subsequent cutting can be taken at 4-5 weeks intervals from mid-November to mid-January and from 3-4 weeks interval onward. This way it gives 50-60 tonnes green forage /ha in 4-5 cuts. In early cuts, the dry matter content may be only 12-14 % but CP may be as high as 16-18%. In late cuts though the dry matter increased to 15-16% but CP goes down to 14-15%. Since, it is a fast growing highly palatable and nutritious legume as well astt enhances the soil fertility so, it is also known as King of the forage crops.

Seed Production

Since, the flowering in Berseem starts from mid-March to first week of April at temperature above 32°C, no cutting should be taken after the end of February or first week of March. Cuttings continue till late produces shriveled seeds under high summer temperature and high wind velocity. Application of seeds setting hormones like Planofix @ 1-2 a.e./litre of water at the flowering stage produces more 9300kg/ha) as well as bolder seeds when the crop is harvested at maturity of the heads. Foliar application of either B-995 or CCC @ 500ppm should also be done to harvest about 35% more seed yield (Yadava, *et al.*, 1978).

Similar to Berseem, another clover, known as Persian clover or Saftal (*Trifolium resupinatum*) as known in India and usually grown in sub-temperate conditions of Himachal Pradesh as well as in some parts of Berseem growing areas, is also a nutritious forage crops but has more water content than Berseem. Some promising varieties like SH-48 and Shaftal-48 have been developed.

Medics (*Medicago species*)

Family: Fabaceae, Sub-family; Faboideae; Genus: *Medicago*

Herbaceous annuals as well as perennials, erect stems with whitish pith, trifoliate with central leaf peteolated, denticulate margin, yellow to violet flowers in short racemes which develop into half circled ring like pods bearing 3-5 kidney shaped seeds of pale yellow in colour. There are about 70 species of which many are weeds and some of them are forages. These are found in Asia, Europe and some parts of Africa. Among the forage species, *Medicago sativa* is the main species grown throughout the world (Photo 22 A, 22 B).

Lucerne/ Alfalfa/Rizka (*Medicago sativa L.*)

Historical Background

Lucerne is originated near Eastern Central-Asia; Transcaucasia, Iran and the highlands of Turkmekistan. Its uses were discovered in Babylonian Text from the year 700 B. C. Since, during first Century, alfalfa was cultivated around Lucerne Lake in Switzerland hence, it is referred to as 'Lucerne' in Europe. From Italy, it moved into Spain and is called "Al'fal'fa means best forage". Latter on in 1578, it was taken to France, Germany and England. From Europe, it was introduced in to America. Since, it is widely grown in South Africa, Australia, New-Zealand, North and South America under diverse conditions and also due to its quality, it is crowned as the "Queens of the Forages".

Soils and Climate

It is a crop of neutral to high pH to slightly saline soils. Though, red laterite soil of low pH is not ideal however, it can be successfully cultivated after neutralizing the acidity through application of lime. Too light to too heavy clay soils are not suitable. Lucerne is grown in some countries below the sea level to an altitude of 2500 m in the temperate to tropics regions of the world. It prefers relatively high temperature for germination. Low temperature during vegetative phase restricts the growth but high temperature results in fast growth and thus days of cutting intervals are reduced.

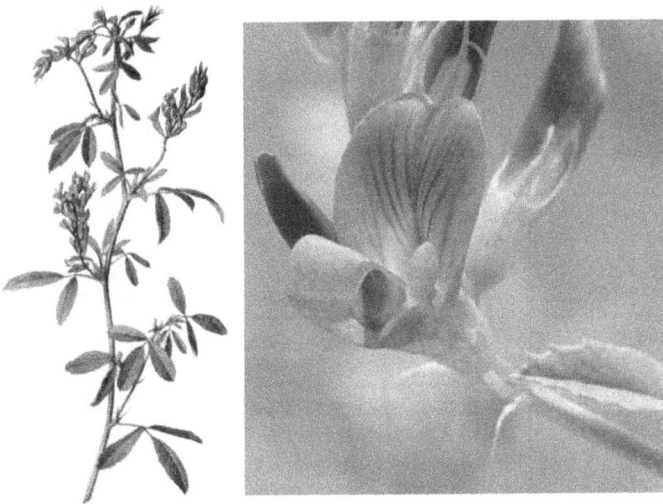

Photo 22A. Lucerne/ Alfalfa/Rizka (*Medicago sativa* L.) *Plant & Flower*

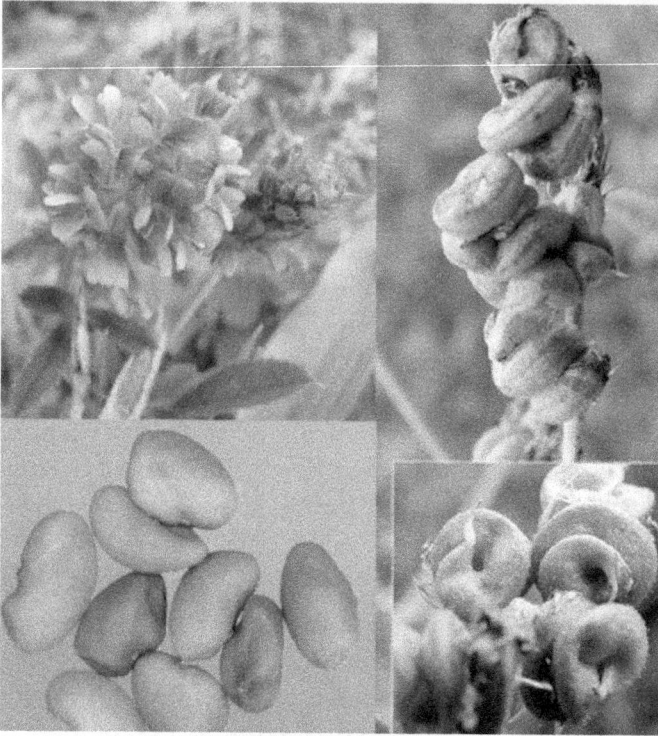

Photo 22 B. Lucerne/ Alfalfa/Rizka (*Medicago sativa* L.) *Flower, Pods and Seeds*

Varieties

Varieties	Characteristics
Anand-2 (GAUL-1)	It is a selection from perennial type grown in Bhuj area of Kutch region of Gujarat, gives 80.0-100.0 t GF/ha in 8-12 cuts. In acid soils of Jharkhand with lime+boron+ Molybdenum gave 11 time more yield (80 t/ha) as compared to control and 3 t seed/ha
SS-627(GAUL-2)	A selection from Sirsa material good for north Gujarat gives 80-100 t GF/ha in 10-12 cuts.
Chetak (S-244)	Selection from single plant local material of Mathura of 70-90 cm height with dark green foliage and light purple flowers. Highly productive and fast re-growth gives 140-150 t GF/ha is excellent for growing elsewhere in India
Sirsa type-8, Sirsa-9 and Type-9	All are developed at Sirsa of medium yielder from 70-80 t GF/ha and better suited in temperate region.
Co-1	An old variety being grown in Tamil Nadu since long is also good for other regions. It is highly protenous with green herbage yield of 80-90 t /ha. Perennial type can be grown continuously for 3 years if protected from rain and weeds during monsoon.

Contd...

Contd...

Varieties	Characteristics
L.L. Composite 3	Selected from 20 clones is fast growing, high yielding germ plasms collected from Gujarat is a low yielder (40 t GF/ha).
L.L. Composite 5	Selection made from 125 downy mildew resistant clones from Kutch for Punjab. It gives 70-75 t GF/ha in 7-8 cuts.`
Lucerne No.9-L	It is a perennial type and remains for 5-7 years in the same field. It has slendrical stalks and bears purple flowers, gives up to 70 t GF/ha
NDRI No.1	A perennial type is a selection from material of Saurastra and Kutch, has deep root system and turgid stems with small leaves can withstand for several years without degeneration. It gives first cut after two months and altogether 100 t GF/ha/year.
RL-88	It is also a perennial type selected from local material of Ahmadnagar can be grown in all region under irrigated conditions. In 10-11 cuts it gives about 100 t GF/ha .
Anand Lucerne-3 (AL-3)	Developed from pure line selection and population improvement of the material collected from Kutch area is a perennial with high branching (45-47 branch/plant) and high yielding (about 100 t GF/ha).

Package of Practices

Alike to Berseem, Lucerne also requires inoculation. The seed treatment is exactly done as it is done in case of Berseem. For this, *Rhizobium melilotii* bacteria containing culture is used. Generally, dry sowing of Lucerne in rows at 25-30 cm spacing with furrow depth of 3-5 cm in well prepared soil is done. About 15-20 kg seeds/ha is required. The irrigation is provided just after sowing if, the soil is dry but in moist soils with medium to high water retaining capacity it may be irrigated after emergence. In winter season irrigation at an interval of 4 weeks while in summer months it may be given at an interval of 3 weeks or even in alternate weeks. One hoeing and weeding after 30-35 days of sowing activates the plant growth.

Nutrients Requirement

Lucerne is a highly nutritious forage crop. Therefore, it requires well fertile soils besides heavy composting. As such, basal application of 10-12 tonnes/ha of well rotten compost + 20-25 kg N/ha + 50-60 kg P_2O_5/ha +25-30 kg K_2O/ha should be done. If, it is to be cultivated in acid soils of pH < 6.2, water soluble boron <0.5ppm, and molybdenum <0.02 ppm, lime @ 2- 3 tonnes/ha should be applied as per soil pH before 8-10 days of sowing and only then FYM and other source of nutrients can be applied. 4-5 kg/ha of Boron as 40-50 kg of Borax and 0.5-1.0 kg/ha of Molybdenum as 1.5-3.0 kg of Sodium-molybdate or Ammonium-molybdate should be applied at the time of sowing to increase the forage productivity by 10-12 times in these soils. (Bhagat *et al.*, 1985; Prasad *et al.*, 1989 and Prasad *et al.*, 1990) A normal plant of Lucerne should contain about 35 ppm of boron and 2 ppm of molybdenum.

Cutting Management and Yields

Nipping of the crop at 5-7 leaves stage activates the growth enzymes and plan growth may be faster as compared to those un-nipped plants. Subsequent cuttings can be available at intervals of 4 weeks during short day length and low temperature below 20°C and at 3 weeks interval during neutral to long day length and high temperature above 30°C. 30-40 cm tall plant can be cut by leaving 4-5 cm from the ground level. It gives more number of cuttings as compared to Berseem. As such, Berseem can produce the herbage only up to first week of April or even at the end of March while Lucerne can supply forage round the year if, proper drainage system is maintained during rainy season. Even in high rainfall area with poor drainage, it can continue to give forage till the start of heavy rain in July. In about 8 cuttings from December to June, 70-80 tonnes /ha of green forage with equally 20-22% of dry matter and CP can be harvested.

Seed Production

Self-pollination in Lucerne is not enough to produce sufficient quantity of seeds. Therefore, cross-pollination by the insects is a must. Since its flowers are tightly enclosed hence, it is difficult for honey-bees to penetrate the same and put the pollen in contact with stigma and style. For this, bubble bees can only trip the female parts and get smeared with pollens to fertilize the same.

The flowers start to appear in last week of February hence, last cut should be taken in at this stage and then the crop should be left for seeds production. Since flowering, pods setting and maturing simultaneously occur hence regular pickings of the pods are required. These plants can be finally harvested before the onset of monsoon and seeds can be threshed dried and packed air tight. This way about 250-300 kg seeds/ha can be obtained.

Spraying of gibberellic acid (0.005%) and indole acetic acid (0.001%) at bud initiation and 50% flowering stages influenced the crop growth and flowering in plants which produced the higher biomass and seeds (Krishna, *et al.*, 2006).

Utilization

Besides its forage values, Lucerne has several medicinal uses including as a tonic to health. It is rich source of Calcium, Vitamin A and D. Alfalfa a homeopathic tonic is very common. In addition to this, according to one report, if, 10-20 seeds of Lucerne are soaked for over night and eaten during the morning helps in reducing the acidity and gas formation in stomach.

Chapter 8

Forage Trees/Shrubs

Several species of trees and shrubs are used as forage especially at the time when there is an acute shortage of common fodder occurs while shrubs and trees some times become the main source of animal feed in arid and semi-arid regions of the world. However, some of the fast growing nutritious shrubs and trees are grown in different part of the world as one of the major sources of forages.

Subabul (*Leucaena leucocephala*)

Subabul (*Leucaena leucocephala*, Lam.De Wit) belongs to the Family: Fabaceae (Leguminosae); Sub-Family: Mimosoideae tribe is a tetraploid (2n=4x=40) leguminous tree/shrub as per management. It is also known with different synonyms viz;

Acacia leucocephala (Lam.) Link
Leucaena glauca Bench
Mimosa glauca sensu L.
Mimosa leucocephala Lam.

In different countries, it has different common names as follows.

S. No.	Common Name	Country
1	Guage	Mexico
2	Koa Haole	Hawaii
3	Ipil-Ipil	Philippines
4	Subabul	India
5	Vaivai	Fizi

Morphology

It is a fast growing leguminous forage tree or shrub which depends on the objective or the purpose for which it is grown. It attains a maximum height of 20m with bi-pinnate 4-9 pairs of pinnae of 35 cm length and 11-22 pairs of 8-16x1.2 cm leaflets. The numerous flowers in globose heads of 2-5 cm, stamens-10, pistil-10mm long, pod-14-26 cmx1.5-2cm green which turns to brown at maturity, bears 18-20 oval shaped brown seeds/pod of 20-25 cm long (Photo 23 A and 23 B).

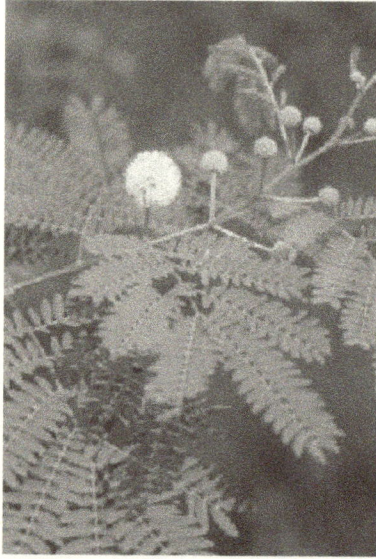

Photo 23A. Subabul (*Leucaena leucocephala*)

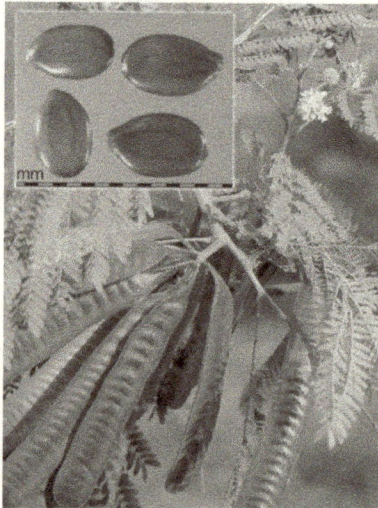

Photo 23B. Subabul (*Leucaena leucocephala*) Pods and Seeds

Physiology

Deep tap root system has characteristic to trap water efficiently since it performs 'di-photonic movement' (It is the movement of the roots in search of water) to sustain under drought conditions. The leaves also perform 'xeric movement'. It is the movement of the two leaflets at right angle so that one leaflet dorsal side is covered by dorsal side of another leaflet to minimize rate of transpiration. It also occurs at the point of photosynthetic saturation during scorching sunlight.

Distribution

Leucaena is distributed in almost all the tropical countries to sub-temperate world to some extent. It is natural vegetation in Yucatan Peninsula and Isothomus of Tehuantepec in south Mexico and widely in tropics. In Philippines, it was identified as a feed for ruminant livestock during 16th century. Presently, it is one of the major forage species in a number of countries where livestock is treated as the major enterprise.

Ecology

Though, it favours hot and humid climate from sea level to 1000m however, it also grows well even at 3, 000 m.s.l. The only difference is that as the elevation increases, the plant height and vegetative growth decrease due to drop in temperature but the seed production is increased due to frequent flowering and seed setting. It gives maximum vegetative growth at 25-30°c temperature and the growth ceases at temperature below 15-16°c. High rainfall (3,000mm) is conducive but it sustains well even in semi-arid to arid highlands of only 650mm of rainfall.

It is grown in a wide range of soils from low to high fertility, from low to high pH (5.5-8.5). Initial growth during the first year in low pH soil may be slow but the growth is stimulated from the next year as the roots penetrate the deeper soil layer where the pH is relatively high. It favours the Ca rich soils and even fit for saline soils.

Cultural Management

Seed treatment is needed to facilitate easy germination of the seeds. The seeds are either treated in hot water at 80°c for 10 minute or dipped in concentrated sulphuric acids for 5 minute and then washed by normal water 2-3 times. The treated seeds are directly sown preferably in line on raised rows at 20-25 cm plant to plant and 1.0 m from row to row spacing. The plantation of saplings raised in polythin tubes is done on the same spacing. For raising saplings, equal mixture of soil, sand and compost is prepared and put in to the 30 cm long and 10 cm diameter tubes in which one seed is seeded in the month of May-June. Water is added as and when required. The 15-20 cm tall saplings are planted during mid-June to July. About 15-20 kg seeds/ha or 50, 000 saplings are required for forage production. In first year, only one cutting of about 80 cm tall plants is taken at 50 cm height in the month of August-September. From second year onwards, 3-4 cuttings during rainy season and 2 cutting during winter-summer months at constant height of 90 cm at an interval of 6 weeks can produce 70-80 tons/ha of green forage with about 20-22% dry matter and 24-25% CP. It has 60-70% digestibility, 6-10% ash, 30-35% N-free extract, 0.8-1.9% Ca and o.23-0.29% P.

Toxicity

Usually, 30-35% of fresh subabul forage to total ration is recommended due to mimosine, a non-protein amino acid toxicity. It has antimitotic and depilatory effects on animals, usually sheep. Young leaves contains 12% while in total it contains 4-5% of mimosine but some new varieties contain less than 2.5% of mimosine which is within the safe zone.

Varieties

Varieties	Country (Year released)	Details
Tarramba	Australia (1995)	Bred by the University of Hawaii from seed collected at 1675 m altitude in Mexico as K636. Establishes rapidly and psyllid and cool tolerant than 'Peru' and 'Cunninghum'
'Cunningham'	Australia (1976)	Bred by CSIRO, Australia is a cross of 'Peru and CPI18228 from Guatemala. Branched, 30% more yield than 'Peru' and good for low temperature area.
'Peru'	Australia (1962)	Brought from Peru to CSIRO as CPI 18614. Branched and more yield than El Salvador cultivar. Good for arid zone of 750 mm RF and temperature >10°c.
'El Salvador'	Australia (1962)	From Hawaii to CSIRO as CPI 18623. Taller (>15m), less branching than 'Peru' easier in germination.
'K8'	University of Hawaii	Arboreal accession during 1960s to1980s. Widely planted in tropics but badly affected by psyllid insect.

Contd...

Contd...

Varieties	Country/date released	Details
'K28'	University of Hawaii	A multipurpose accession prior to K636 and good for acid soils.
'LxL'	University of Hawaii (1996)	Developed from 5 k series clonal interspecific *L. leucocephala* F1 hybrids. Good for subtropical conditions.
'Romelia'	Colombia (1992)	CIAT 21888 selected at La Romelia, 2,700 mm RF, 1,400 msl, soil pH 5.1 and Al saturation 22%.

Uses

Besides, its uses as a forage crop, it is also used in raising soil fertility, fuel purposes, as timber, in preparation of pulp and paper as well as extraction of resin from seeds for fibre in textile industries.

As such;

— One kg dry wood of Leucaena gives 1600 BTU of heat which is equivalent to $1/3^{rd}$ of the heat given by 1 kg of natural gas.

— An established crop fixes about 500-550 kg N/ha/yr, is the highest N fixation by any legume.

— Seeds are also used as food in some of the countries.

— Decoxiation of bark is used as a family planning measure.

Since, it has multipurpose uses hence, it is declared as a 'Wonder Tree' by the USDA.

Shevri (*Sesbania sesban* L.)

Sesbania or Egyptian riverhemp is a member of Fabaceae (Leguminiceae) family having 236 genera and 17 species. It is a narrow crowned, deep rooted multistemmed tree or shrub of 4-8m height. Leaves are bipinnetely compound of 2-8cm long with 6-27 pairs. It performs well between 200-500m elavation from high humidity to arid conditions. The height and vegetative growth are slow and low at high altitude but seed production is high. The long thin pod bears several seeds. The seed size is about half to Leucaena seed hence, 8-10 kg seed/ha is required. It is generally grown in marginal rocky soils on the fences. It is a good range species for saline-alkaline soils in arid and semiarid regions. The Agronomy for growing this species is almost similar to subabul. The yield and quality of the forage is not as good as Leucaena (Photo 24).

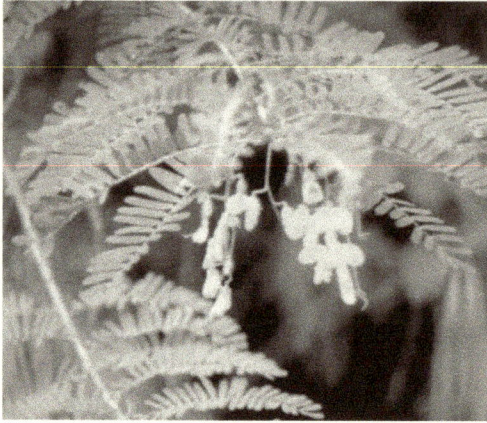

Photo 24. Shevri (*Sesbania sesban* L.)

Acacia (Acacia tortilis)

Acacia tortilis or Israeli Babool is native to Savanna and Sahel of Africa (Sudan) where it is known as Umbrella Thom as a fodder tree for the desert. Out of 135 species, 4 (*A. tortilis, A. albida, A.senegalensis and A. Arabica*) are common as a forage shrub/tree. It belongs to Kingdom: Plantae, class: Magnoliopsida and family: Fabaceae: tetraploids (2n=4x=52).

Morphology

Plant height to 21m, leaves 2.5cm in 4-10 pairs of pinnae upto 15 pairs of leaflets, flowers small of white colour and aromatic, spring like coild pods consisted of tight cluster flat seeds (Photo 25).

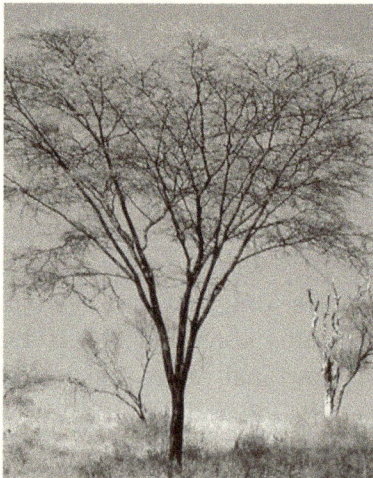

Photo 25. Acacia (*Acacia tortilis*)

Soil and Climate

It is a very drought resistant plant for the deserts of saline to alkaline soils conditions which can sustain in very low to extremely high temperature (0°-50°c). The areas receiving even 40mm of rain fall to as high as 1,000mm are good for its growth. In deserts, it is an excellent for plantation on the sand dunes to rocky scarps. It is introduced in Rajasthan (India) in 1958 and grows twice faster to indigenous species.

Cultural Practices

The seed are scarified and treated in hot water (80°c) for 5-10 minutes or treated in sulfuric acid for 15-20 minutes. The seeds are directly sown in the field in1-2 cm deep holes or planting of the 3-5 months old 400 seedlings/ha is done during rainy season. These seelings are grown in 30cm long polythene tubes. The cuttings are taken after 2 to 3 years of full grown trees.

Importance

In Indian desert, a full grown tree can give about 25 kg green forage/tree/year. Forage leaves and pods contain 12% digestable protein and seeds with 38% CP. It also gives 6.1 MJenergy/kg of dry matter and also helps in producing good quality of honey. In addition to that, it has timber, tannin, gum and medicinal values. Its umbrella like top structure gives shelter to animals during scorching sun light.

Insects and pests

Under extreme desert conditions, 90% of flowers are dropped. Bruchid beetles can destroy about 90% of the seeds. Another, Buprestid beetle (*Julodisy* sp.) defoliates 50% of green leaves and Post beetles (*Sinoxylon* sps) changes felled timber to dust in a week.

Chapter 9

Plant Population Dynamics

Succession theory as well as grass and tree phenology_together establish the plant population dynamics.

1. Succession Theory: Succession is the orderly process of community, change in which one association of species replaces another. In other words, one type of vegetation succeeds or follows a preceding or former type into the said area.

It may be of two types:

1. **Natural succession:** It happens under climax conditions, either due to change in soil caused by flood or change in vegetation due to severe drought.

2. **Induced succession:** It happens due to human interference causes severe erosion and finally changes in natural vegetation.

Natural change in vegetation occurs under arid or extreme rainfall conditions, resulting in flood. The change in vegetation also occurs due to change in soil-water retaining capacity as well as its fertility and weeds infestation.

The soil development is the function of several factors;

Soil f cl, o, r, p, t

Where; cl, is climate; o, is organism; r, is rellief or topoghaphy and exposure; p, parent material and t, is time, taken in soil formation

Since, soil is a function or product of climate, organisms, topography, parent materials and time of its formation hence, changes in any one of these parameters, induces a change in the soil development.

As the soil has direct relation with its vegetation hence,

V f cl, p, r, o,t Where, V is any property of vegetation that expressed in quantitative term.

Besides these, temperature, precipitation and stipness of the topography are the other factors, govern succession.

Stages of Succession

Initial or pioneer stage → Transition stage → First herb stage → Climax stage

These stages of succession in soil and vegetation can be expressed as under:

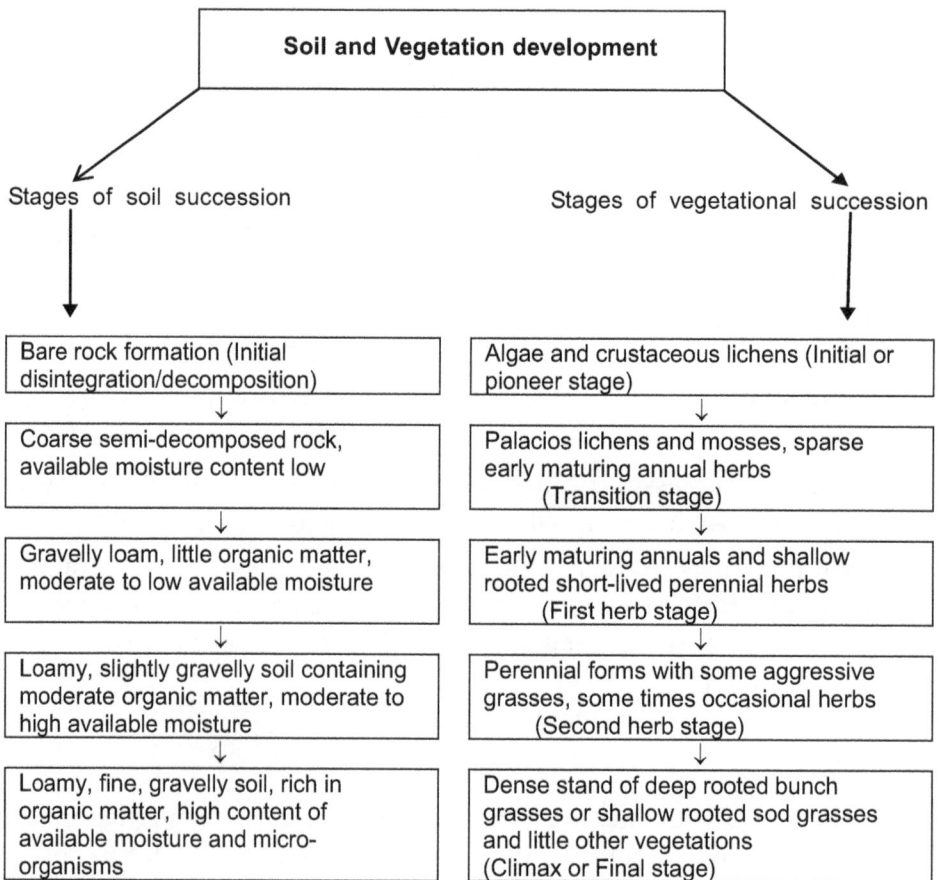

Soil and Vegetation development	
Stages of soil succession	**Stages of vegetational succession**
Bare rock formation (Initial disintegration/decomposition)	Algae and crustaceous lichens (Initial or pioneer stage)
Coarse semi-decomposed rock, available moisture content low	Palacios lichens and mosses, sparse early maturing annual herbs (Transition stage)
Gravelly loam, little organic matter, moderate to low available moisture	Early maturing annuals and shallow rooted short-lived perennial herbs (First herb stage)
Loamy, slightly gravelly soil containing moderate organic matter, moderate to high available moisture	Perennial forms with some aggressive grasses, some times occasional herbs (Second herb stage)
Loamy, fine, gravelly soil, rich in organic matter, high content of available moisture and micro-organisms	Dense stand of deep rooted bunch grasses or shallow rooted sod grasses and little other vegetations (Climax or Final stage)

Fig. 9.1 Soil and plant succession/development, where grass is the final climax in well developed soil

2. Grass and Tree phenology/Variation in growing period: It is another parameter which establishes the plant population dynamics. Since, vegetational phenology differs from plant to plant and season to season hence, grazing system/period is managed as per plant growth. It varies on;

a. Land situation (high land to low land)

b. Rainfall pattern and total rainfall

c. Soil topography and types

d. Soil fertility status and nutrients application

e. Vegetation types and their growth habit

f. Regeneration potential of vegetation at frequent cutting/grazing

Therefore, grazing is decided on the readiness of the ranges or regeneration capacity under the different soil and climatic conditions

Chapter 10
Grassland Distribution

Rotation of the earth results shift in the path of the sun over the earth surface to tilt the polar axis on either sides of the North and South equators at 23° 17′ angle and area between 0° – 23° 17′ on both sides is known as tropics and from 21° 17′ to 35° on both sides is sub-tropics. About one fourth of the land surface and two fifth of earth's total surface lie between tropic of Cancer and tropic of Capricorn, receives about 50% of the world total rainfall. Since majority of temperate and tropical vegetations occur from 0° to 30° hence it is also known as "biological boundry" .This zone also shares one third of the world population These tropics and sub-tropics (A-C) and temperate to polar (D – F) with the following characteristics Trewarth, 1954-68) in which types are indentified with capital letters and subtypes with small letters.

A. **Tropical humid climate** – Hot and humid with 750-1000 mm rainfall and scorching sunlight covers 20% land area and 43% of sea surface.

   Ar. Tropical wet (rain forest) – astride the equator from 5-10° latitude either side has uniform high temperature and heavy rainfall for 10-12 months.

Aw. Tropical wet and dry (savanna) – extending beyond 20° latitude: lower rainfall, less well distributed and less reliable than in Ar.; shorter wet and longer dry season, may continue to 9 months.

B. **Dry climate** – Only occurs over land surface and boundry fixed by rainfall, evapotranspiration more than precipitation; extends from equator to tropics and into the middle latitudes, covers about 26% of the continental area. (Fig. 10 2)

   Bs. Semi-arid or Steppe – Little rainfall, highly variable and irratic, just south of Sahara desert covering major parts of Ehiopia and Sudan (Africa).

   Bw. Arid and Desert – Almost no rain and occational drizzling over a very limited area stress to life.

C. **Sub-tropical climate** – Occurs in middle latitudes except tropical mountains; seasons distinguishes as wet and dry since temperature continue over 10°c for 8-12 months with little fluctuation.

   Cs. Subtropical dry summer known as Mediterranean – seasonal rainfall of dry summers and humid winters, warm to hot summers, mild winters covers about 1.7% of earth surface.

   Cf. Subtropical humid – occurs on eastern side of the continent has hot summers with rainfall, mild winters with frost and occational snow.

D. **Temperate Climate** – Lying beyond 40° latitude; divided into milder oceanic and more severe continental climates.

E. **Subarctic climate (Boreal)** – extended towards pole beyond 50° latitude.

F. **Polar climate (Tundra)** – Occurs in the higher latitudes of Tundra and ice cap.

G. **Highlands** – found any where except Australia with difficult to identify the types of climate.

In addition to above climatic classification, some others have also classified the climate in different ways. Among these, Troll (1965) classified the zones, based on vegetation has practical utility for the selection of species adaptation into.

1. Polar and subpolar zones
2. Cool temperate zones
3. Warm temperate zones and
4. Tropical zones

It is in more detailed than Trewarth but boundaries of major types are almost similar in which tropical Africa and South America were identified on the basis of rainfall of the wet – dry period as under:

Zone	Humid months	Arid months
Belt of tropical rainforest and transitional woodland	12- 9.5	0-2.5
Humid savanna belt	9.5 - 7	2.5-5
Dry savanna belt	7- 4.5	5-7.5
Thorn savanna belt	4.5 - 2	7.5-10
Semi-desert belt	2 - 1	10-11
Desert belt	1 - 0	11-12

Climate and Grasslands

True grassland is an open tract of land consisted of dense cover or tall or short grasses and associated herbaceous species devoid of or scattered shrubs and trees. Different terminology is used for different types of grasslands in different countries. In South Africa, grasslands are known as dry, Highveld and montane types. In Kenya grasslands situated between 2200 - 3000 m with minimum of 1000 mm rainfall are known as highland grasslands while in Ethiopia grassland above 2 500 m with 750-1275 m elevation is termed as Montane open grasslands. In Australia, Tussock and Hummock grasslands of subdesert are known as steppe.

In several regions open grassland is replaced by grass-woody plant associations. In East Africa canopy cover is measured for sharing of trees and shrubs to grazilands where grass dominated lands with less than 2% scattered trees and shrubs are known as grasslands. The grasslands of the world are broadly classified into Savannaha to Desert and Alpine grassland as latter is independent of any other types. The sequential event of the development of first type can be summarised in brief as under:

Savannah: (Scattered woodland + Tall coarse grasses without turf)
Tropical or subtropical climate. Example: Llano of Venezuela, Campo
of Brazil, High-grass & tall-grass savannas of Africa

↓↑

Prairies: (-Trees + Unpalatable sod-forming tall low productive grasses)
Warm or cool climate of deep, dark, fertile soils. Example: Trans-
Mississippi Valley, the great Black Earth Belt of Ukrainia &
Humid pampas of Argentina

↓↑

Steppes: (-Trees – tall grasses + sod-forming short-grasses + few legumes)
Semiarid or arid, warm or cool climate. Example: Great Plain of US
East of Rocky Mountains & Southern Russia

↓↑

Scrubs: (Dominated by thorny plants with very few grasses)
Arid region or periphery of the worlds' deserts

↓↑

Deserts (Absence of vegetation with a few thorny unpalatable plants)

Sequential degradation and improvement of Grassland types of the world

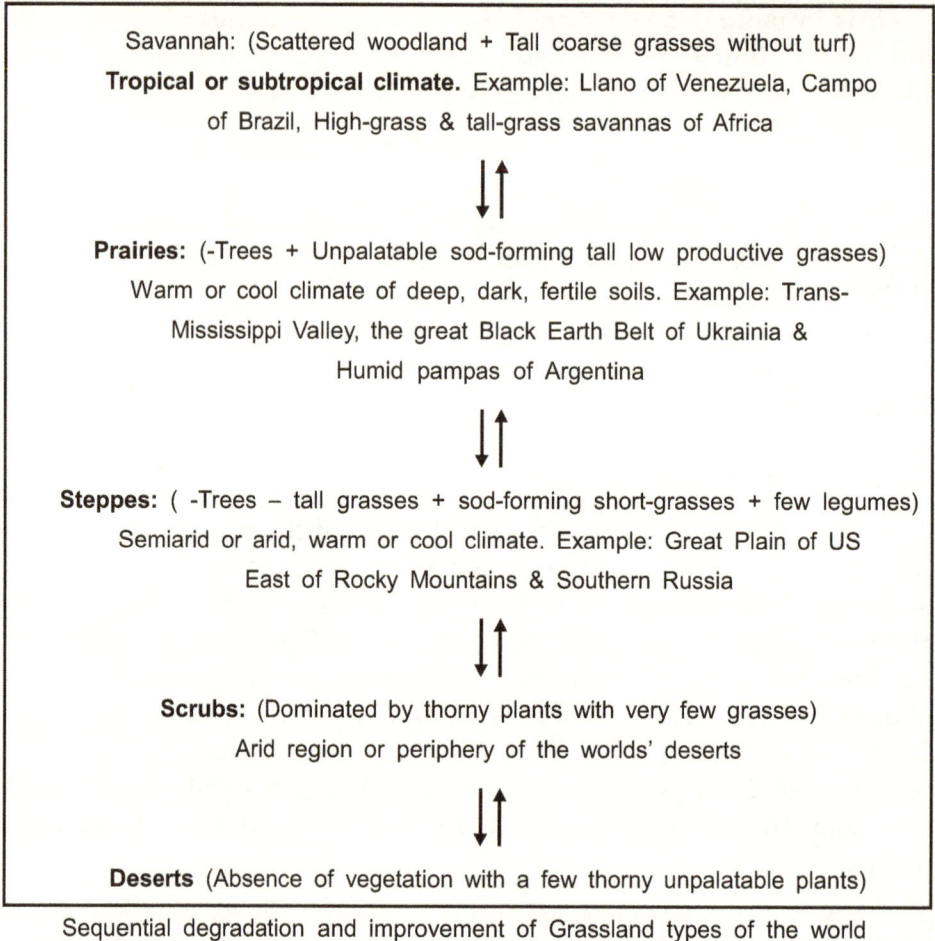

The above figure is the gist of different grassland types of the world with their soil types and main vegetation. As such the Savanna/ Savannah (derived from a Spanish word 'Zavana', meaning grass covered treeless plain) grassland is the top final type of vegetation with scattered woodland and tall grasses found in hot humid and high rainfall regions of south-west of African continent and Venezuela and Brazil of South America. The degradation or devoide of woodland, facilitates the development of Prairies with unpalatable sod forming tall grasses. It is developed under both warm and hot climates. The deep dark fertile soils are the main characteristic of this grassland. Mississipi Valley, the great Black Earth Belt of Ukrainia and Pampas of Argentina are the some classical examples of such type. The further product of the sequential events, is the formation of true grassland type, Steppe which is dominated by palatable sod-forming grasses and legumes.It is primarily found in semi-arid, warm and cool climates. Great plain of North America and south Russia, east Australia and central Africa are the true grassland (Steppes) types of the world.The extreme exploitation of the Steppes grassland gives birth to Scrubs which is further deteriorated to deserts.

Further protection to desert and elimination of scrubs followed by introduction of promissing genotypes of vegetations, helps in renovation of the grasslands from Steppe to Savannah. Since grassland is the event of serial development as such over exploitation of the resources results in formation of desert and proper management helps in renovation to an initial status.

The savanna or savannah grassland is further grouped into 5 types by Cole, 1963.

1. Savanna woodland; is the deciduous woodland of tall trees (> 8 m) and tall mesophyte grasses (> 80 cm) where the spacing of the trees are more than the diameter of the canopy

2. Savanna parkland: is a combination of tall mesophytic grassland (> 80 cm) with scattered deciduous trees (< 8 m height).

3. Savanna grassland: is the tropical grassland without trees and shrubs.

4. Low tree and shrub savanna: is the widely spaced trees plus low growing perennial grasses (< 80 cm height) and

5. Thicket and scrub: is the trees and shrubs association without stratification.

Alpine

Alpine grassland is an Independent of the above types which is found nearer to both the poles after tundra as well as highlands (above 1,500 m.s.l.) of different continents. In India, it is found in low rainfall (375mm) Chini area of Himachal to high rainfall (3750mm) area of Darjeeling, perennial grasses like, *Chrysopogon gryllus, Phelum alpinum* and *Poa pratensis* are the dominant species. Among annuals, *Poa annua, Oryzopsis lateralis* and *Polypogon fugas* are common. Presence of conifers tall plants which are also in abndence in highlands of eastern Africa sub-temperate conditions, identify the semi Alpine types of vegetation. The most economical forage legumes like Clovers and Medics are supposed to be the gift of Alpine grass cover.

Indian Grasslands

Indian grassland is classified both on the basis of climate by Trewarth, (1954-68) and on the basis of vegetative covers by Dawadghaw and Narayanan (1972).

Climatic Regions of India

On the basis of climate, the Indian grasslands have been classified in to seven types from desert to tropical wet (Fig. 10.1)of which three of them are large in size that covers more than 75% and the rest four occupy less than 25% of geographical area.

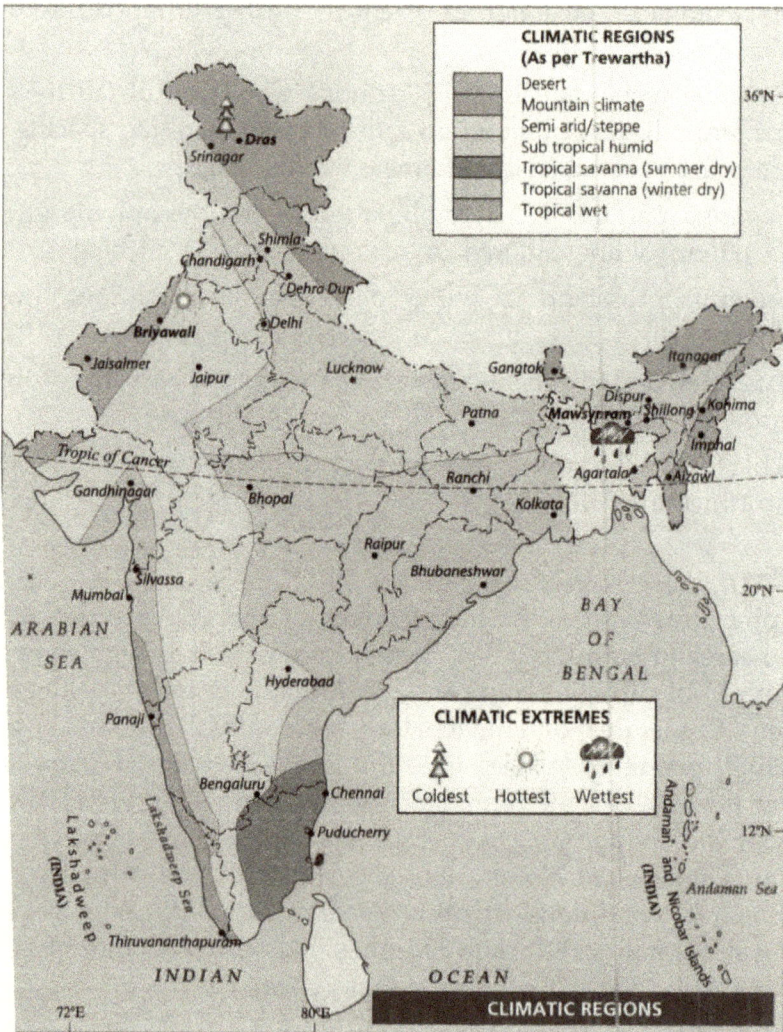

Fig. 10.1. Climatic regions of Grasslands of India

Grass Cover of India

Indian grasslands is a product of shifting agriculture, cutting of forest trees, over grazing and burning and hence, no one is an out come of climatic climax. Whyte, (1964) categorized the Indian grasslands of four types, found in tropical and subtropical regions. Latter on Dawadghaw and Narayanan (1972) illustrated the different stages of succession of these grass covers including Temperate and Alpine Cover of Himalayan in the North and Nilgiris in South.

1. *Dichanthium—Cenchrus—Elyonurus* **Cover**: This type is found in North-west arid and semi-arid regions having alluvial to sandy-loam soils between 23°N latitude and 60-70°E longitude of Punjab, Rajasthan, U P and North Gujarat. Almost all the important grasses are found in this region but it is being deteriorated due to un-controlled grazing. Such process can be controlled as illustrated under.

Stages of regressive and progressive successions due to grazing and protection:

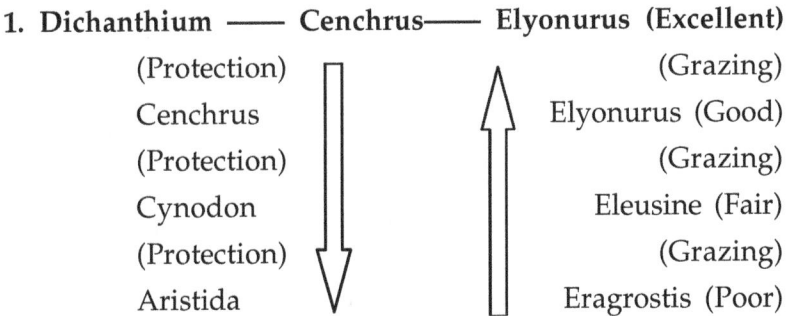

1. Dichanthium —— Cenchrus—— Elyonurus (Excellent)

(Protection)	(Grazing)
Cenchrus	Elyonurus (Good)
(Protection)	(Grazing)
Cynodon	Eleusine (Fair)
(Protection)	(Grazing)
Aristida	Eragrostis (Poor)

2. *Sehima — Dicanthium* **Cover**: The hilly undulating terraces with gullies and valleys comprises of Deccan and Jharkhand plateau extending from Madhya Pradesh, Bundelkhand region of U.P., Chattisgarh , Jharkhand and South Rajasthan with red to black soils are covered with majority of perennial grasses.

Regressive and progressive successions as caused by burning, erosion, grazing and protection, respectively

Sehima   Dichanthium

(Excellent)

(Burning)   (Erosion) (Grazing)   (Protection)

(Moisture)

Cymbopogon

                                                                 Iseilema

Ischaemum

          Themeda *Pseudanthistiria*   *Bothriochloa* (Good)

                    Chrysopogon   (Protection)

(Grazing)

                    Heteropogon   *Eremopogon* (Fair)

(Grazing)   (Protection)

Aristida—— Eragrostis——Gracilea (Poor)

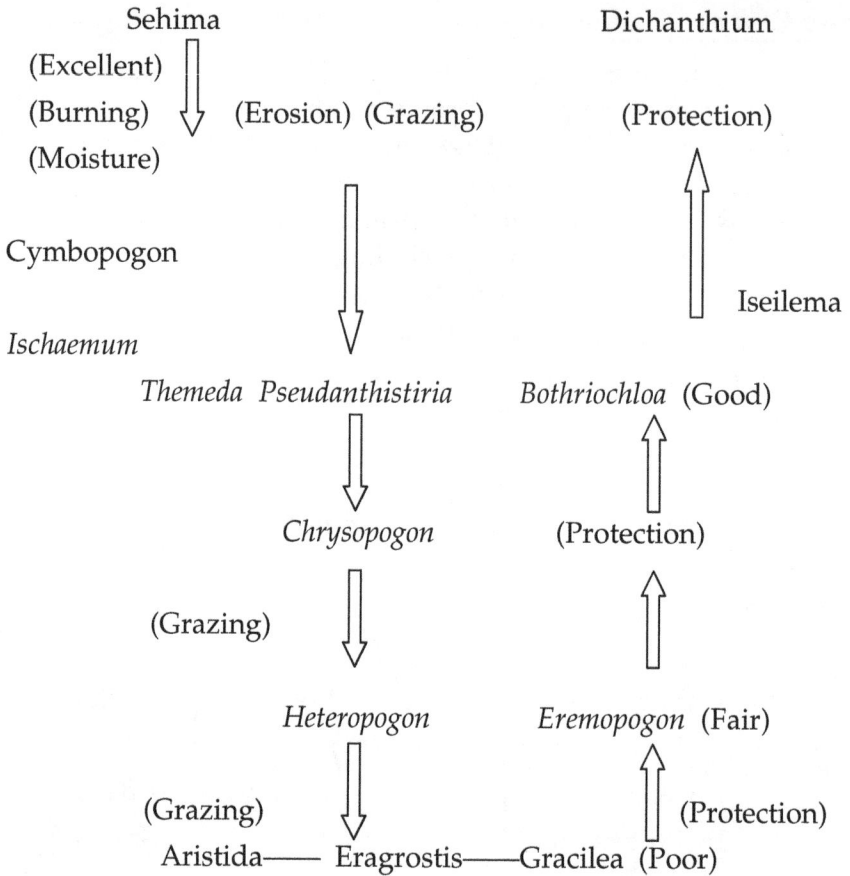

3. Phragmites — Saccharum Cover: This cover is found in North-East humid region of India in the basin of the Ganges and Brahmaputra. It is characterized by low-lying, ill-drained soils due to high water table comprises of tall, coarse unpalatable grasses, used for thatching.

4. Themeda — Arundinella Cover: This is found in hilly region of Northern mountain belt at 500 to 2500 m elevation of which *Themeda anathra* is the dominant species and *Heteropogon—Eragrostis* is the degraded form.

5. Temperate and Alpine Cover: Grass cover of Himalayan and Nilgiris regions is identified by different temperate grasses including some very important forage legumes like medics, vetches, white and red clovers

Grasslands of the Continents

Distribution of plant associations in which grass is the dominant partener of the vegetation is of two types (10.2)

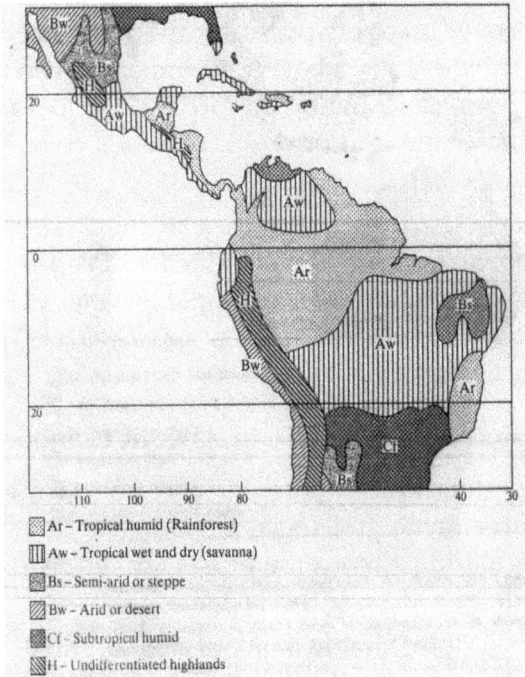

Ar – Tropical humid (Rainforest)
Aw – Tropical wet and dry (savanna)
Bs – Semi-arid or steppe
Bw – Arid or desert
Cf – Subtropical humid
H – Undifferentiated highlands

Fig. 10.2. Koeppen's world climate (Trewarth's 1954-68)

1. Association of savannas grasslands, woodlands and shrub forming natural communities and

2. Areas modified to produce grazinglands

Grassland of Africa

The majority of African grasslands are found from humid forest area of Congo basin and along the coast of Western Afica woodland savanna with sparse grass cover. (Fig. 10.4) These can be categorized as:

1. **The high-grass savanna (high grass low tree):** This is present in tropical rain forest of Congo basin. 15°N. *Andropogon*, Blue stem grasses, *Pennisetum* spps., Congo signal, sorghum and millets of 3-4m height are the dominant vegetation.

2. **The tall-grass savanna (Acacia-tall grass):** This is found in east and south parts of Africa is situated at 8 °N of Sudan and highlands

of Ethiopia (Montane open grasslands at about 2500 m and upward, under 750 to 1275 mm rainfall) Uganda and Kenya. *Andropogon* spps., *Themeda* and *Hyparrhenia* of 1-1.5m height are the main habitat. Here, mountain grasslands or temperate-type vegetation cover associated grasses are dominant where as *Setaria* and *Pennisetum* associated with savanna or woodland vegetation is usually presence. Moving towards 12°N to Indian Ocean, the rainfall reduced and arid or desert region is covered with *Panicum, Cenchrus* and *Chloris*.

3. The tall-grass (high veldt) prairies of the Transvaal and orange-free state developed under temperate climate. Deep dark brown fertile soils (Vertisols) are the classical example of this prairies grassland. *Aristidia spps.*, Rhodes grass, Natal grass and *Digitaria* sps. are the main grasses found in this prairies.

Importance of Forages and Pasture in African Economy

Agriculture system of a country or a region is the product of the interaction of soil, climate and social custom. The livestock production or forage/ rangeland management has an edge over food crops production in Ethiopia due to the fact that:

1. Among the 68% of arable land of the country, 54.0% is under Forage, Pasture/Range system and thus only 14% is under food crops production. This might be due to

   (a) low rainfall followed by low water retaining capacity of the soils together with low soil fertility, do not facilitate high input requiring food crops and thus comparatively more resistant crops say, growing of grasses and legumes are the better option of which livestock is the best consumer

   (b) Majority of non-vegetarian diet may be the other dominating factor for rearing of livestock as such livestock: human population ratio is >1 in Ethiopia as compared to other African countries.

Hence, the livestock sector vis-à-vis forages production is more sustainable, is playing better roles in Ethiopian Agriculture system.

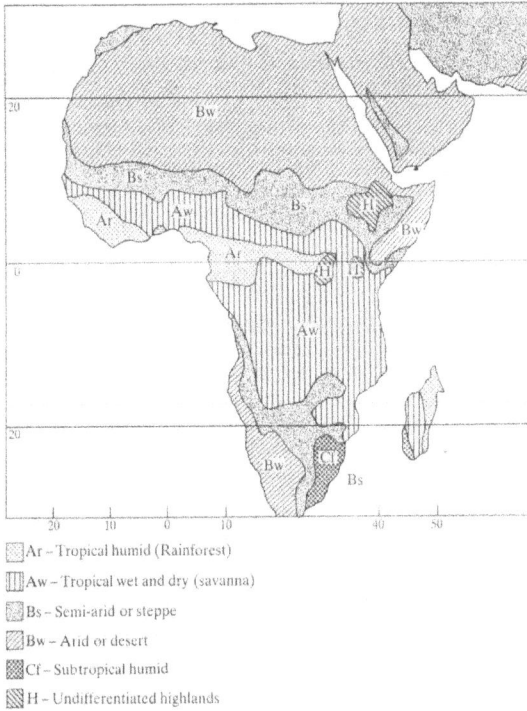

Ar – Tropical humid (Rainforest)

Aw – Tropical wet and dry (savanna)

Bs – Semi-arid or steppe

Bw – Arid or desert

Cf – Subtropical humid

H – Undifferentiated highlands

Fig. 10.3. Koeppen's world climates (Trewarth's 1954 and 1968)

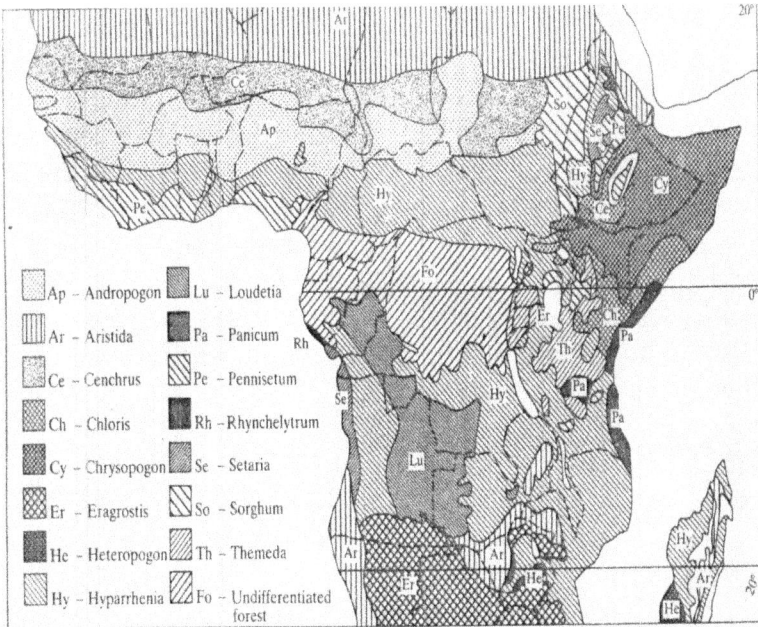

Ap – Andropogon
Ar – Aristida
Ce – Cenchrus
Ch – Chloris
Cy – Chrysopogon
Er – Eragrostis
He – Heteropogon
Hy – Hyparrhenia

Lu – Loudetia
Pa – Panicum
Pe – Pennisetum
Rh – Rhynchelytrum
Se – Setaria
So – Sorghum
Th – Themeda
Fo – Undifferentiated forest

Fig. 10.4. The grass cover of tropical Africa.

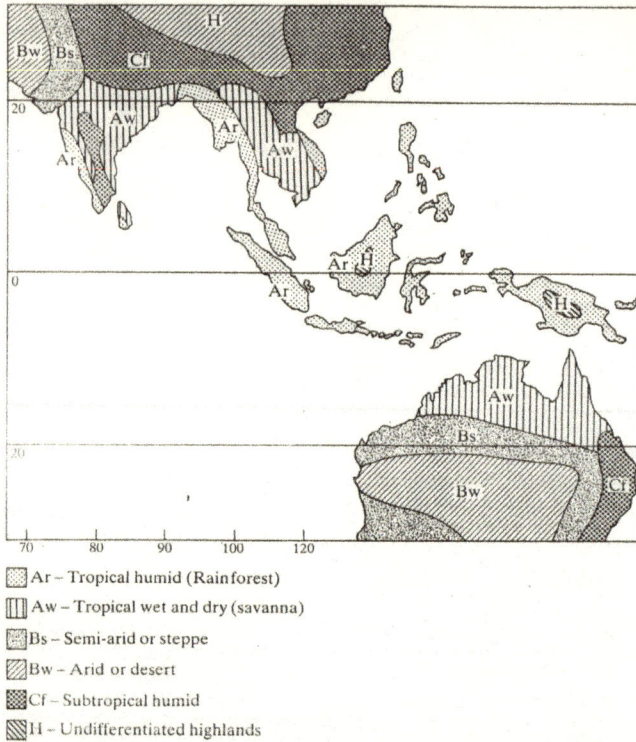

Fig. 10.5. Koeppen's world climates (Trewarth's 1954 and 1968)

Though, major part of the land area is under range system however, the carrying capacity of these rangelands is very low. As such in Australia, where 5 Animal unit (AU) is maintained on 1 acre of pasture in contrast to Ethiopia where, 5 acre rangeland is maintaining 1 AU only. Thus, availability of forages to livestock industry is far from adequacy alike to several developing countries. Therefore, improvement in productivity of such rangelands is the only way out to enhance the production potential of livestock which directly influences the socio-economic conditions of the farmers; as a result it has a direct bearing on the national economy.

Grassland of South America

The great natural grassland of South America (Fig. 10.5) is one of the largest grasslands of the world extended from Patagona in southern Argentina passing to southern and central Brazil through Uruguay. Warm season grasses such as *Andropogon, Paspalum, Panicum* and *Eragrostis* are found in the north.is termed as **campos** are consisted of a treeless savanna and a sub-division (*campo cerrado*) with scattered tree and bush savanna. The second one is **"The Great Amazone basin"**, a tropical rainforest with association of *Panicum* and *Paspalum* grasses and *Stylosanthes* and *Desmodium* legumes. The third one is the Vast Grassland of *llanos* extending from Colombia to east-north Venezuela to the Atlantic Ocean with scattered palms savanna

North America

Prairie stretches from central highlands of Mexico where sparse grazing land with arable crops at water points are found. Much of the north-west

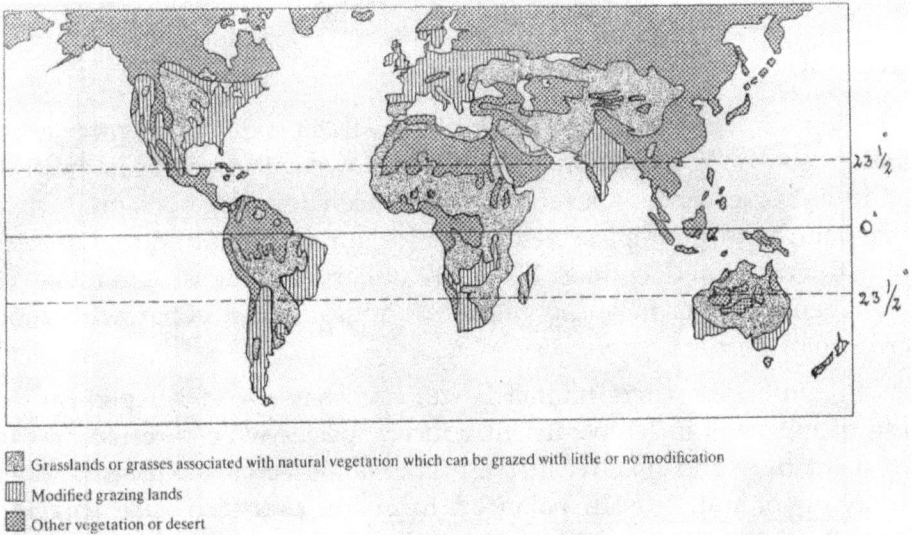

Grasslands or grasses associated with natural vegetation which can be grazed with little or no modification

Modified grazing lands

Other vegetation or desert

Fig. 10.6. Major grazing lands of the earth (Moore, 1966)

Mexico, is desert savanna that has been replaced by woody vegetation along with various species of cactus and *Yacca* have created serious problems for range management.Therefore, a very small area of this continent is under grassland Tropical grass species of *Andropogon, Cenchrus, Setaria, Panicum, Agrostis* and *Prosopis, Agave, Accasia* shrubs with *Mimosa* are the dominant species.

Europe

Eropean grassland is composed of improved grasses and legumes (10.6). Around the Mediterranean a dwarf tree-shrub climax is known as **Chapparal** has been changed by heavy grazing.

Asia

Asian grasslands from India to S-E Asia extending upto Papua and New Guinea are the outcome of high humidity, high rainfall and high temperature with few exceptions. Among these grasslands, the Indian grasslands has been classified under different grass-cover have been already discussed in this chapter. In addition to Grass-cover of India, Sri Lankan grassland is a wet and dry-zone grassland while S-E Asian grassland is an open and mixed grasslands composed of scattered tree savannas with majority of tropical grasses and legumes. Short grassland (upto 60 cm tall), mid height (1.5 m) and tall trees above 1.5 m height is the combination of Papua and New Guinea grasslands (Fig.10.5).

Australia

Though, very large area of central Australia is desert however grass and grass-woody formation in the north (Townsvill) to nort-east tropical and sub-tropical zones (Queensland) have been developed into productive grassland with the replacement of native species by introduced species of both grasses and legumes. These are under semi-intensive to intensive management with balanced nutrient application on a par with food crop management.

In south-east where rainfall is sufficient has also developed by the use of nutrients in temperate introduced species which are the best in both quantity and quality. In these grasslands aerial broadcasting and spraying of nutrients in balanced form are practiced. The carrying capacity of the grassland is very high (5 A.U./ Ac) as compared to sub-Sahara Africa (0.2 A.U./Ac). That is why more than 70% of Australian National economy is from the advanced Dairy Industries.

Chapter 11

Pasture Management

Pasture Establishment and Renovation

Pasture

Pasture is an artificially managed/established land of grass(s) with legume(s) on which the domestic animals are grazed on rotational/ controlled basis.

Pasture Establishment

Pasture establishment is defined as the sequence of events that occurs from time to time, the seeds are sown until such time that the species are in a position to contribute substantially or permanently to pasture production.

The establishment of pasture depends on various factors from region to region or, from savannah to arid as well as alpine conditions. Thus it depends on monsoonal climate (duration, number of rainy days and intensity of rainfall.

1. Soil types with their physico-chemical properties
2. Temperature, latitude and altitude
3. Types of ecology and natural vegetation
4. Live stock population and types as well as demands between foods and forage crops or, say competition for land between man and animal.

Establishment of Pasture on a Virgin Land

It depends on:

1. Land situation
2. Choice of pasture types/systems
3. Soil fertility conditions and evaluation
4. Selection of species as per soil and climate

1. Land Situation: The points to be taken under consideration are:

a. A virgin land where soil erosion is a problem; species with well developed root system to bind the soil as well as having a dense canopy structure to cover the soil to give protection from rain should be preferred

b. If, the initial fertility of the soil is poor, legume should be preferred as a preceding species.

c. A pasture can be developed on good fertile soils if, countries having dairy as their main source of national income.

d. If, there is a degraded forest land: development of Agroforestry like Silvipasture, Hortipasture can be preferred.

e. Watershed management with creation of lakes and ponds is a must to control soil and water on one hand and recycling of water on the other.

f. Plantation of trees or creation of shades for cattle should be made.

2. Choice of Pasture Types/Systems: The types of pasture to be developed will depend on their objectives and duration.

No.	Types	Objectives	Duration
1	Permanent pasture	High soil fertility with Dairy as a main source of economy	Several years without ploughing
2	Long duration pasture	6 years perennials followed by 2-3 years annuals	6-10 years
3	Short duration pasture	3-5 years perennials followed by cash crops	4-5 years
4	Temporary pasture/Leys	Annual legumes to raise soil Fertility for succeeding food crops	1-2 years

3. Soil Fertility conditions and Evaluation: The soil physical conditions and their physicochemical properties must be assessed before establishment of a pasture and possible correction should be made, accordingly. Preferably, the selection of the grass-legume species may be done as per soil conditions. The following parameters should be under taken.

a. Soil physical properties: Soil depth, structure, texture, water retaining capacity at 1/3 rd bar to 15 bar and organic matter (%) should be assessed.

b. Soil chemical properties: Soil pH, status of essential macro and micro-nutrients for plants as well as toxicity of Fe, Al and Mn in general and of heavy metals (Pb, Hg, Cd and Ar etc.) in particular should be analyzed.

4. Selection of species:

I. Species must be adapted to the soil and climatic conditions for that potential local species should be preferred over exotic or introduced one.

II. Species must be suited to the purpose/objective of the pasture.

a. If, the main objective is to improve the soil fertility hence, the proportion of legumes with high nitrogen fixing ability should be more in proportion to grasses.

b. Livestock; Composition of mixture should be palatable, nutritious as per choice of the heard.

c. Lean period consideration: Species may supply green herbage during scarcity period say, during drought and flood

d. Soil erosion control: Species should have well developed root and canopy structure to check soil and water erosions.

III. Companion species must be compatible to:

a. Both species should response well under one management system

b. They should be equally competitive

c. Equal in regeneration capacity after each grazing/cutting

d. Ease in seed production or availability

e. Species may be ease to establish, persistence and tolerant to drought and

f. Longer vegetative growth period.

Establishment of Sown Pastures

Sown pastures are the improved grazing lands comprised of introduced and / or legumes for temporary or permanent grazing systems. Such pastures can be established by

1. Improvement of native or natural grassland sods through nutrients addition and introduction of potential new species local or exotic through seeding /planting.
2. Renovation of a previously developed pasture which is being deteriorated.
3. Development of previously cultivated land if, dairy is preferred above food crops
4. Development of degraded forest land
5. Renovation of problematic soils through introduction of resistant genotypes.

The following steps will be needed for the establishment of pastures in above situations.

Land Preparation

If the land is very undulating, levelling to a possible extent with cleaning, weeding, terracing and ploughing etc. will be done

Soil analysis

For an ideal productive pasture, status of soil physical and chemical conditions must be assessed and species may be selected, according to their acidic or alkaline conditions as well as their water holding capacity along with sufficiency or deficiency of a particular nutrient. Thus, optimization of the nutrients is extremely needed for a balance soil-plant-animal system.

Seed Treatment

For an early normal stand of the grass-legume species proper seed treatment after germination test for fast germination and other for inoculation of legume seeds facilitates optimum growth of the species. The hard seed coats either need scarification or hot water treatment. It may also be treated with sulphuric acid for 5-10 minutes as per hardness of the seed coat. If, it is legume, it is further inoculated with its specific bacteria.

Methods of Sowing

The sowing of seeds can be done with different methods as per situations. In a large area, mixing of the grass: legume seeds in 50:50 or 75:25 ratio can be done. In smaller area, either dibbling or line sowing is preferred for ease in further operations. Row ratio is adjusted on the basis of prior experiments since it varies from location to location. Therefore, the said association may give the maximum production to per unit area with economically and biologically sustainable together with an improvement in soil fertility.

Nutrients application

Basal as well as annual monitoring of the nutrient in soil-plant system gives stability in production potential of the pasture system. Therefore in addition to initial status and application of desired nutrients, optimum level of the nutrients in soil and plants must be assessed at least once in a year or at the beginning of the rain or active growth period of the species.

Weeding and Cultural Operations

Mechanical weeding should be preferred over the chemical weeding in a pasture system to avoid slow poisoning and pollution of the environment. If, there is an advent of irrigation, the land may be watered. This will allow the weed seeds to germinate. As soon as the weeds fully germinated, the land should be ploughed down to destroy the weeds. This may be also done if, it rains after the land preparation.

Grazing Management

An efficient grazing management is the prime need for a sustainable pasture system since over grazing is the main cause for deterioration of the pastures. Therefore, a manager must take an account of the following parameter.

a. Grazing Capacity: Grazing capacity or, Carrying capacity is the number of animals given to a pasture to support at a given time or, for a period of time or say it is the ratio of **Animals/Time.**

b. Stocking Rate: It is the number of animals to per unit land area or, a ratio of Head or **animal/Area** (ha or ac).

c. Grazing Pressure: It is the number of animals per unit of available herbage or, ratio of feed demand to feed supply (**Herbage yield/ Animals).**

Therefore,

$$\text{Grazing Pressure (GP)} = \frac{(\text{DM demand}/\text{Animal day}) \times \text{No. of Animal unit}/\text{ unit area}}{\text{DM availability}/\text{day}/\text{unit area}}$$

If, GP > 1, means over grazing

GP < 1, means under grazing

GP = 1, means balance grazing or, = Carrying capacity

Yearling Unit/ Animal Unit:

YU/AU = 1 adult cow + her 6 months old calf

Or, = 1 horse or, = 4-5 goats/sheep's

Systems of Grazing

1. Deferred Grazing: Deferred grazing is preferred in a pasture system having an association of perennial grasses and legumes in which provision of both seeds and herbage is made. The pasture land is divided into 3-4 sub-blocks or paddocks as bellow:

A	B	C	D
Deferred for seed production in 1st year	Grazing alternatively ------------------→	--------------→	--------------------→

In 1st year, A paddock is deferred for seed production and grazing is allowed in rest of the paddocks alternatively. As such, in 2nd year, B is deferred for seed and grazing is done in others. Thus, C and D are deferred in succeeding years. Thus, the seeds produced in one paddock are used for seeding in all the paddocks. Hence, it gives equal opportunity for reseeding. Such pastures give less nutritive herbages due to perennial species.

2. Rotational Grazing: This system is followed for a pasture developed with annual plus perennial swards. Here the land is divided into 4 sub-blocks (paddocks).

A -------→	B -------→	C -------→	D

←---

The grazing is allowed in these sub-units on systematic intervals so that flowering may not initiate. Since, there is no provision of seed production is made hence, each year reseeding is done to maintain proper population. It provides more nutritious forages due to annuals and grazing before budding.

3. Deferred-Rotational Grazing:

1st Year	I	II	III
2nd Year	III	I	II
3rd Year	II	III	I

I to III denotes the year in which it is deferred.

It is the combination of both deferred and rotational systems of grazing in which perennial species are kept to maintain the population. The pasture is usually divided into 3 paddocks. Alternatively, each paddock is given chance for seed formation after allowing grazing till 1/3rd period of vegetative phase of the main species and then left for seed production. Thus, in first year, grazing is allowed only for 1/3rd period of vegetative growth and then deferred for seed formation however, grazing is continued in II and III. Subsequently, paddock II is deferred during second year and paddock III during third year in the same fashion to that of first. Since, provision for both seeds as well as herbage is made hence the system is called as such.

4. Hohenheim System: This system of pasture management and grazing is an improvement over the rotational system. This had been developed by Hohenheim of Germany after the World War II when there was a huge scarcity of forages in Europe. Under this system, the pasture is divided and the animals are graded as high, medium and low milking. First, high milking animals are allowed to graze for few days, followed by medium and low producing. The pasture is maintained under fully irrigated conditions along with high rate of nutrients. It is the fastest system of grazing in which annuals species of grass –legume dominates over perennials. It provides high and nutritive forages in which provision of seed production is hardly made hence, seeds are to be procured every year.

5. Strip Grazing: It is followed to increase the milk productivity by allowing the milking cows to graze only within the limited fence of highly vegetative patches by putting low voltage electrical bars in front and behind the animals. The low producing animals are allowed only to graze what ever left by the predecessors.

6. Continuous or Free Grazing: This system is practiced in arid and semi-arid regions with large paddocks and animals. These pastures are poorly fenced. Grazing is controlled by water supply. In good season, stock numbers are increased and in a bad season, surplus animals are sold or slaughtered. Over grazing allowed the inferior plants to come out resulting in degradation of pastures. Extreme exploitation of soil and plant resources without addition of any input resulted in serious consequences of desertification of the grazing lands.

Ley Farming

It is a grass-legume sward explicitly (clearly/openly) sown as part of a predesigned rotation of crops, the intension being to plough-up again after a pre-determined number of years.

1. Very short term leys: 1-2 years

2. Short term leys: 3-4 years

Thus, ley is an integral part of a crop rotation/sequence and is designed ultimately to be ploughed up, so it is regarded as a pivotal crop on which our rotation is based,

Objectives

1. To build soil fertility for succeeding crop

2. To provide nutritious forage to livestock

3. To increase the productivity of succeeding food crops.

Establishment of Leys

The establishment of leys depends on the types of grass cover of the region, from steppe to alpine types with consideration of the following factors:

1. Intensity and duration of rain

2. Natural vegetation of the region

3. Cattle pressure and competition for land between food and forage crops as well as forestry

4. Soil physico-chemical properties

5. Soil topography, elevation and temperature round the year

6. Consideration for humid to arid conditions

Steps to be taken

A. Choice of Land and its preparation:

1. A virgin land susceptible to erosion

2. Fertility status of soils

3. Fertile soils if, dairy is the main interprise

4. Degraded forest land

5. Problematic soils

B. Corrections of mineral deficiency and and reclamation: Problematic soils (Acid soils, Alkaline soils, saline and Water logged soils)

C. Provision of Terracing, levelling, cleaning, weeding, drainage and others operations

Maintaining Soil Fertility

Since main objective of 'Ley farming" is to use it as a preceding vegetation to enhance soil fertility for the succeeding food crops hence, the following steps should be taken to meet the objectives

1. Grazing by sheep on rough grasses and folding them at night

2. Keeping adequate legumes population

3. Ploughing down of legumes if, they are in excess

4. Grazing may be preferred over cutting

5. Grasses of well developed root system be preferred to break crum structure.

Some good results of leys as a preceding crop and cereals as a succeeding crop have been reported from tropical as well as from temperate countries.

Chapter 12

Range Management

Rangeland: It is a large, naturally vegetated area of relatively low productivity, mostly unfenced, graze by livestock and race animals. It is native to the area.

Or, it is uncultivated grasslands, shrub lands, or forested lands with herbaceous and / or shrubby under story, particularly those areas producing forage for grazing or browsing by domestic and wild animals. (Vallentine and Sims, 1980).

1. Range management and Range Improvement

Scientific range management: is based on the premise that vegetation can be used perpetually for grazing while simultaneously providing with high quality air and water, open space and recreation (USDA, Forest Service, 1970).

Range management is the care of natural and semi-natural grazing lands. More technically, it is the manipulation and utilization of rangeland soils, vegetation and animals for production of goods and services needed by man (Heady, 1975).

Range management is an art and science of planning and directing the use of rangelands to obtain optimum, sustained returns based on objectives of land ownership and on the needs and desires of society (Vallentine and Sims, 1980).

The above definitions entail to manage the naturally vegetated areas of palatable herbs, shrubs and trees as a livestock feed on a sustained basis.

Most of the rangelands of the arid and semi-arid regions of the world are unfenced areas with sparse grass vegetation which is a product of un-controlled grazing system and finally on the verge of extinction due to extreme exploitation of the natural resources. Under the circumstances these are now extending in to desert like situation which needs urgent renovation.

2. Characteristics of Rangelands

All continents of the earth have extensive arid and semi-arid lands which are classified as range lands (Gonzalez, 1969).having the following characteristics

1. Rangelands receiving rainfall < 750 mm or some times higher having soils and topography unsuitable for cultivation
2. It produces timber and provides watersheds.

Among the different continents of the world, Australia with 69% of its total area is as a rangelands and livestock farming, is the main source of national economy (Table 12.1).

Table 12.1: Continents and Area (%) Under Rangeland

Continents	Area (%)
Australia	69
Africa	51
Eurasia	29
America	15

A large tract of land of South America and African countries is under rangelands (Table 12.2).

Table 12.2: Area Under Rangelands

Countries	Area (m/ha)
Argentina, Brazil, Peru and Venezuela	300
Ethiopia	65
Kenya	87
Uganda	60
Tanzania	50
S. Zimbabwe	90

3. Principles of Range management

The rangeland has two principles to manage it effectively.

1. Associated with animals
2. Associated with vegetation

1. Principle related to animal practices: It has the following points to be taken for consideration:

   a. Grazing intensity/stocking rate to keep balance between production potential of the land and and number of animal until (AU) that can grage so that the herbage is neither wasted nor destroyed

   b. Control over kinds of different values for man

   c. Proper distribution of animals to avoid over grazing to check the deterioration in vegetation and soil erosion

   d. Animal grazing as per season/plant growth pattern.

2. Principle related to range management: It relates to Agronomical management of the rangelands which includes:

   a. Weed control and proper use of fire if, essential

   b. Seeding/planting of potential forage species to fill the loss of natural vegetation

   c. Nutrient assessment to control soil fertility for optimum productivity

   d. Incorporation of organic source of nutrients to maintain soil physical and chemical properties

   e. An efficient watershed management for efficient re-use of rain water to control loss of soil and water.

4. Causes of Rangeland deterioration

There are several reasons for deterioration in rangelands of arid and semi-arid regions of the world. All these are due to extreme exploitation of natural resources or better to say Biotic – Climax rather Climatic – Climax. These may be due to;

a. **Over grazing:** due to heavy pressure of animal on unit land

b. **Climatic changes:** prolong drought due to environmental pollution resulted in extinction of palatable species

c. **Uncontrolled fire:** Burning to control weeds some times leads to un-control fire and vast devastation.

d. **Shifting in cropping patterns:** High pressure of human population enforced to put more and more land under food crops and thus caused pressure on range system

e. **Communal grazing:** no control on number of animals and duration of grazing leading to fast deterioration in grass cover.

f. **Socio-economic conditioned:** Number of cattle keeping is assumed as a status symbol, whether well managed or not

g. **Soil erosion:** Heavy grazing leads to severe nature of soil erosion resulted in loss of top fertile soils and vegetation

h. **Incidence of rodent and predators:** some times damage to plant roots by rabbits, hares and rats etc. also causes serious loss to vegetation.

5. Range Conditions and Assessment

It is the departure in the botanical composition of the rangelands. It indicates the amount and stability of the herbage and reflects quantity (a measure of stocking rate) and quality (a measure of out put)It can be graded as under:

a. **Excellent:** 75 — 100% carrying capacity due to an excellent mulch

b. **Good:** 50–75% carrying capacity due to bare spots and some soil erosion

c. **Fair:** 25–50% carrying capacity due to infestation of weeds, more bare spots and gully erosion

d. **Poor:** < 25% carrying capacity due to water and wind erosions and severe loss of mulch.

6. Appraisal of Range Conditions

Production potential of a range can be assessed by improvement or deterioration which requires a technical knowledge of the following indices;

a. Desirable plant species must be equally competitive under one soil, climate and management conditions

b. Species should be accepted by the animals

c. Infestation or aggressiveness of weeds is an indicator of deteriorating conditions of the rangeland

d. Deterioration in soil fertility reduces the productivity as even, deficiency of one essential nutrient result in 80% loss in yield.

There are some approaches to assess the range conditions:

A. Quantitative – Climax approach: Here, comparison of the present vegetation with previous composition from undisturbed patches is done by assuming it as 100 % and thus, the present conditions of the range in question can be graded as:

a. Increaser (%)

b. Decreaser (%)

c. Invador (%)

There may be increase or decrease in the above two component species but increase in the invader or say, weeds is an indicator for deterioration in range conditions. Therefore, the adjustment in stocking rate and their distribution can be done, accordingly.

B. Qualititive – Rating approach: Under this, palatability of the component species along with their nutritive value are assessed before putting the animals and the range is graded as excellent to fair

C. Range – potential approach: The comparison of the present botanical composition to that of last year or before the grazing is done and is graded in the similar fashion as excellent to good or fair and from fair to poor, accordingly.

D. Score- card approach: Under this approach, the conditions of plant species, soil and animal performance are evaluated as:

a. General growth and vigour of the species

b. Density of the component species and over all their grazing value

c. Composition of annuals, perennials, grass and legume, weeds and poisonous plants

d. Soil erosion indicators *i.e.,* extent of mulch and types of erosion

e. Animal productivity to per unit area.

1. Grazing System as a Management Technique in Rangelands: Management of ranges is almost similar to pasture system particularly as far the grazing and reseeding are concerned. The frequency of grazing depends on the frequency and total rainfall. As such, the carrying capacity of well managed Australian rangeland is 4-5 animal unit/acre as compared to 5 acre land is required to rear only one animal unit in free grazed poorly managed sub-Sahara African rangelands.

Under Indian desert conditions in long term seasonal grazing of Lasiurus-Eleusina-Aristidia cover Sharma *et al.* (1980) recorded an overall improvement in perennial species vegetational cover from 11.1 to 77.7 per cent in 7 years due to better soil and periodical rainfall.

Burning as a management practice: Large areas of rangelands are repeatedly burnt every year either with planning, mistake or due to natural causes. Fire has a greater and more direct influence on bush encroachment and herbage productivity of various grazing lands than any other method used for bush control. Though, Scientists oppose the burning since it directly influences air pollution however, it has the priority to manage the rangelands.

Advantages of burning

1. Burning as a tool for shifting agriculture
2. Controls undesirable plants, mainly bushes
3. Remove the over matured un-palatable stems
4. Obtain more desirable species composition such as *Panicum maximum, Andropogon gayanus, Heteropogon contortus* as they are tolerant to burning and seeds of *Stylo* species a in general and *S. humilis* in particular are tolerant to burning as these are escaped through mixing in soil
5. Stimulate growth out of season and improve herbage quality
6. Facilitate easy movement of livestock, helps in uniformity in excreta distribution
7. Kills serious pests and reduces chances of diseases
8. Prepares an ideal seedbed to facilitate easier germination
9. Adds nutrients in general and K in particular

Disadvantages of burning

1. Burning causes deterioration of vegetation
2. Results in a drastic reduction in reserve materials of roots and crowns
3. Increases erosion due to creation of open surface devoid of vegetation
4. Loss in organic N, organic matter and other minerals since, they would have been added if, they would have been incorporated in the soil as green manure
5. Some times, uncontrolled fire leads to national problem
6. It increases air pollution

Time, Frequency and Intensity of Burning

Burning to every 3rd or 4th year is sufficient to control bushes. Burning just at the time when trees are sprouting but grasses are still dormant is preferred. An intense but rapid fire is desirable.Burning reduces the organic matter and increases the pH of the rangeland soils but its effect on soil nutrient status is hardly influenced (Vinod Shanker, 1978).

Range Reseeding and Fertilization

If, the plant population is not enough to provide a good soil cover, reseeding may be done after selecting the proper species just before on-set of monsoon or rain. Nutrients application should be done on the basis of their optimum level in soil and plants. Generally, nutrients in terms of organic and inorganic sources are applied as basal or in split preferably just after rain.

Consideration for Seeding/Reseeding

The species may have the following characteristics:

1. Ease to establish
2, Stand maintenance
3. Forage usability in a season / year
4. Season for maximum growth
5. Sustain to grazing
6. Palatable to different animals
7. Optimum nutritive value
8. Biologically competent in association
9. Seed production capability
10. Hay making quality
11. Response to nutrient, water and weed suppression quality
12. Fast regeneration capacity
13. Year round forage supplying quality
14. Free from diseases and pests
15. Stability in yield in different years

Fencing

Fencing is the key tool for establishment as well as for sustainability of a rangeland to control undesired grazing and proper growth of the component species. As per availability of the fund, either trenching or bund with biological fencing by plantation of thorny species can be done. The use of barbed wire or chain fencing may be costly but it gives more protection and prolongs for a number of years.

C hapter 13

Forage Preservation

The preservation of forages is done either when it is in surplus during the main growing season or as a reserve material to be fed during lean periods or during natural calamity; flood and drought. Availability of excess forages during the growing season also gives the option to preserve the forages for lean periods.

Such forages are usually preserved in two forms:

A. Hay

B. Silage

A. Hay

Hay making is the process in which initial moisture of 70-90% of herbages is reuced to 10-15% which contains less than 20% CP and more than 18% crude fibre.

Types of Hay

Based on the technology, the following types of hays can be prepared.

a. Traditional type in which forages are cut and dried withot chopping and stored in small bundles.

b. Here chopped forages are dried and stored and hence it requires less space to store as compared to above one.

c. After drying the bales are prepared with hand followed by compression from machines.

d. Hand –trussed hay is manually made preferably of high nutritious legumes through rapid drying by passing hot air blowing in closed chamber on large scale is also known as barn-dried hay.

Principles

It should be dried very fastly to avoid nutrients loss and as a rule 5% moisture is needed for pelleted cured hay, 10-15% for chopped hay and 15-20% for long stemed loose hay. Swath surface drying is the best for drying in which air circulation as well as radiation remain at the maximum.

High quality hay is prepared from fine-stemmed grasses and legumes cut at right stage; 50% flowering/ milking stage or before maturity in a process so that it never loses any of nutrients during drying. Excellent quality hay may have the following characteristics:

1. It must contains leaves
2. It should be free from mould weeds
3. The green colour must be present
4. It must have pleasant smell and aroma

Crops suitable for Hay making

Thin-stemmed and leafy grasses which may remain palatable and nutritious after drying such as Bermuda grass (*Cynodon dactylon*), *Cenchrus ciliaris, Dichanthium* spps., *Setaria sphaceolata, Heteropogon contortus* and *Bromus inermis* are some of the species of which good hay is prepared.

Among legumes; Clovers to be cut at full bloom stage while Lucerne at half-bloom stage, the other vines producing legumes may be cut at pod initiation stage.

Precautions

1. It should not be cut late or at maturity
2. It should not be dried in open sun light
3. It must contain 75 to 80% dry matter

Hay can also be prepared by drying artificially from hot blower. The fresh material is chopped in small bits and passed through rollers to crush the stems and culms then it is dried in chambers at 20°C to 25°C for a short time. This facilitates in maintaining the nutritive value of the hay.

Methods of Hay Making

On the basis of quantity of availability, weather conditions and facility at hand the hay is prepared by the following methods.

Field curing- is the traditional method followed by the farmers in which the forage is cut and left in the same field or transferred to some other dry places if the field is not dry. The forage is regularly turned till the desired moisture (15%) is not reached. However in acid soil it can not be done due to high infestation of termites which damages the herbage completely.

Barn Drying

It is done on large scale in which the forage is partially dried (40-45%) in the sun and then put inside the barns in rows. Hot air is passed till 75-80% dry matter is obtained, usually after one to two weeks. By this method a minimum loss in quality is achieved.

Dehydration

Dehydration or artificial drying is followed on commercial basis in which chopped material is dried in oven or any other dryers. Generally, highly nutritious meal of lucerne and clovers is prepared to feed poultry and other birds.

Losses in Hay Making

Major loss can occur under high moisture conditions or weting in faulty storage. If the moisture will be high, the fermentation loss will be more while long stay in sun light may cause oxidation and loss of vitamin A. In legumes hay loss of leaves is very common which can be minimized by careful handling during turning and provision of store house at the nearest. Weting of hays due to rain causes bleaching and fungal attack results in huge loss of carotene, protein and sugars. In addition to these losses in quality may also occur due to conservation practices (Table 13.1)

Table 13.1: Nutrients Loss in Hay Process (%)

Conservation Process	Dry matter	Starch equivalent	Digestible protein
Dried on the ground	21	42	34
Dried on appliances	18	39	29
Barn drying	15	35	25

Application of Propionic acid @ 10g/kg water (3 kg/t of 30% moisture containing forage) protects from molds. In dry straw use of urea is also recommended but some time feeding of urea treated straw increases the uric acid of the blood resulted in death of animals.

Weather condition is very important for hay making. It is difficult to cure in rainy season, the time during which excess of forages is available. For this situation, it can be only done under the roof. Comparatively hay making is easier in winter months and to some extent in hot summer under the shade.

B. Silage

Green forage was preserved in Germany in 19th centuary. It gained momentum in 1877 after the publication of a book by French agriculturist, Auguste Goffart of Sologne near Oreleans who given the word as silos. It then moved to USA, UK and other countries.

Silage is fermented, high moisture (50-60%) stored forage. Scientifically silage is the product of both aerobic respiration at the early stage followed by anaerobic fermentation of green plant materials in latter stage and the process of making silage is termed as ensilingor silaging

It is an ideal practice for humid region where hay making is comparatively difficult due to absence of bright sunlight. It is also superior to hay as nutrient loss in silage preparation is also less than the hay.

Crops and their Stages for silage making

Crops containing more sugar are excellent for silage making. As such, sugarcane tops, maize and hybrid Napier are supposed to be the best but some sweet sorghum types as well as Sudan grass are also good for this purpose. Among legumes; Lucerne, clovers, cowpea, soybean, rice bean, sunhemp and vetches are used. Other materials like; vines of sweet potato, peas and beans, surplus fruits and their pulps improved the quality of the silage.

Crops	Stage of cutting
Maize	Milk to dough
Teosinte	Boot stage
Sorghum and Bajra	50% flowering
Oat	50% flowering to dough
Hybrid Napier	1-1.25m tall
Deenanath grass, Guinea grass and Setaria grass	Before ear emergence
Natural grasses	Early flowering

Methods

1. Cut the crops at right stage

2. Cut the forage in 2-3cm long pieces

3. Maintain the adequate moisture to 65-75%

Silo pits may be either cemented pits or towers with side doors at different heights for filling and taking out of prepared silage. In tower system; the cut forages is blown into by blowers. It is well trapped so that maximum quantity of air must be removed and quickly covered. The sealing is also done by putting a layer of 20-25cm sawdust with a little water.

In pits system; the pits are dug at the high locations. These may be a cemented structure or even earthen usually where there is no termite infestation. It is prepared as per availability of the material; as such about **400kg** of forage can be kept in **per cubic m** space.

Filling of the Silo-pits

1. Put 15-20 cm layer of dry rice / wheat straw or dry grass in the bottom

2. Put 25-30 cm layer of cut forages grasses/ cereals :legumes (3:1)and press well so that maximum quantity of air is expelled out

3. Add 10 kg molasses and 1 kg salt to per 1,000 kg of material

4. Again put the another layer of material and repeat the process till 1m above the ground surface and make a dome like structure

5. Put a layer of straw and thick layer of wet clay soil at the top

6. Finally cover it with a plastic sheet to ensure protection from rain

Changes in Fermentation

Aerobic bacteria + yeast + moulds

Green forage $\longrightarrow$ CO_2 + 27-38°C + Lactic, acetic & butyric acids + alcohol

$$\text{If, 65-75 \% moisture + sugar} \xrightarrow{\text{Respiration}} \text{Excellent silage}$$

$$\text{If, protein (\%) higher} \xrightarrow[\text{Anaerobic}(Clostridium)]{\text{Anaerobic lactic bacteria}} \text{Butyric acid formation and moulds (bad silage)}$$

Therefore, to control the Clostridium bacteria the following preservatives / q of green matter is recommended.

Silage Material	Preservatives and/ or Additives
Grasses only	2.7 to 3.6 kg molasses or 4.5 kg citrus pulp / q forage
Grass + Legume	3.6 kg molasses or 4.0 kg citrus pulp / q forage
Legume only	4.5 kg molasses or 6.8 kg citrus pulp / q forage

Among the chemical preservatives, Na-meta-bi-sulphite @ 400 g/q of forage is applied.

Characteristic of Good Silage

Good quality silage has the following qualities

1. Pleasant odour with taste
2. Lactic acids (%) higher means a good silage
3. Light-brown colour is good, dark-brown is fair and black is a rotten one
4. Butyric acid formation means bad silage

Therefore based on the criteria of odour, colour, pH and concentration of fermentation products during enciling, the silage may be of following types.

Criteria	Very good silage	Good silage	Fair silage
Taste	Acidic taste	Acidic taste	Butyric acid taste
Butyric acid	Absent	Traces	More
pH	3.5-4.2	4.2-4.5	4.8
Lactic acid	1-2%	-	-
NH_3-N% of total-N	< 10%	10-15%	20%
Colour	Greenish-brown	Dark-brown	Black

Chemical Changes in Ensiled forage

In presence of oxygen, aerobic respiration takes place for a short period. *Escherichia coli* and *Aerobacter aerogenes* are the two bacteria produce acetic acid from sugars which prevents the putrification. As the temperature rises due to CO_2 formation, the bacteria activated and utilizes the carbohydrates to produce CO_2, and other organic acids (lactic, acetic and butyric acids with a little quantity of alcohol.

Proteins hydrolize to amino acids but under poor conditions this acid is further broken to produce amines. Presence of Ca, Na, Mg and K in forage form salt with lactic acid and volatile acids. Action of organic acids on the chlorophyll gives brown colour and the aroma is due to the combination of acids with alcohol.

Precautions

1. Maintain Grass/Cereal: Legume ratio in 3 : 1
2. Moisture content from 65-75 % by adjusting grass and legume
3. Press well to expel air to maximum
4. Maintain temperature between 28-35°C
5. Add preservatives to maintain quality
6. Maintain the pH from 3-4
7. Maintain the moisture by adding dry and green forages

Even after due care some loss of nutrients in process can not be ruled out.

Table 13.2: Nutrient losses in process (%)

Conservation process	Dry matter	Starch equivalent	Digestible protein
Ordinary	17	32	38
Stimulated	17	22	18
Acidify	13	25	14
Inhibited	17	30	49

In addition to this, about 7-35% loss of silage in various biological processes is estimated.

Advantages of Silage

1. It can be prepared any time in the year which is not possible in case of hay making
2. More nutritious and tasty than hays
3. No shattering, bleaching and leaching losses
4. Higher digestibility than hay and dry forages
5. No wastage of feeds even coarse material changes in to digestable forms
6. Even weeds are utilized with main forages

7. Being a partially digested feed require less energy in digestion by animals

8. Easy in long distance tranport

9. Feed intake capacity of animals is increased and

10. It is a boon for animals generally scarcity of feeds during flood and drought.

Chapter 14

Grass: Legume Associations

**Mixed/Intercrop Associations of Forage: Forage and Food:
Forage species**

Mixed or intercropping of grass/cereal with legume is definitely a biologically and economically sustainable system in terms of maximum exploitation of natural resources. It facilitates in maximization of biological yield with an economically viable system along with supplies a nutritious food and forages in addition to maintain or even improvement in the soil fertility and therefore, it is a more environmentally sound system.

Willey (1979) and latter on other workers have also proposed some biological and economic parameters to evaluate the mixed stands either mixed cropping, intercropping or mix –intercrop associations. Its importance in case of grass-legume associations in rangelands, pasture as well as in cultivated species has significant application in interpreting the result. Accordingly, the assumptions were made that;

Yaa = Pure stand yield of species A

Yab = Mixed stand yield of species A

Ybb = Pure stand yield of species B

Yba = Mixed stand yield of species B

Assumptions:

1. Yab + yba > Yaa or, Ybb

2. Yab + Y ba = Full yield of A + some yield of B

3. Yab + Yba > Yaa + Ybb

Out of the 3 assumptions, the first 2 hold good but there is hardly any possibility of the third. However on the basis of computation of data of several experiment, a fourth assumption stood true. It gave the convincing result that in the mixed stand, both the components species individually produced less than 100% yield in mixed stands as compared to their respective sole stands but over all result was more than 100 % or say, Land equivalent ratio (LER) > 1.

Biological/Competition Functions of Association

1. **Land Equivalent Ratio (LER):** It is the ratio of the mixed stand yield to pure stand yield in same unit of land or it is the percentage yield of one component as compared to yield of same component in pure stand.

   $$LER1 = \frac{Yab}{Yaa} \text{ and } LER2 = \frac{Yba}{Ybb}$$

   Where, LER1 is the partial Land Equivalent Ratio of component A and LER2 is the partial Land Equivalent Ratio of component B

   Or, LER = LER1 + LER2 or, in (%) it is LER1 x 100 + LER2 x 100

   Therefore, the criteria is that LER must be > 1 or, > 100% can only be accepted .

2. **Competitive Ratio (CR)**

   It is the ratio of the LER1 : LER2

   The CR ratio should be = 1 or say, both crops are equally competitive

   If, Cr > 1, means component A is more competent than B and if, Cr < 1, means component B is more competent than A

3. **Aggressivity (A)**

   It is the difference between the 2 partial land equivalent ratios.

   Or, LER1 – LER2 = +, - or, 0

   If, it is (+) means A is aggressive over B and

   If, it is (-) means B is aggressive over A

   If, it is = 0, means there is a cohesiveness between both the species and the same is the most acceptable association.

4. Crowding Coefficient (CC)

It also indicates as which one species is dominant and which one is recessive from their respective crowding coefficient and is represented by K1 and k2 as;

$$K1 = \frac{Yaa - Yab}{Yab}; \quad K2 = \frac{Ybb - Yba}{Yba} \quad (\text{ For 50 : 50 ratio })$$

$$K1 = \frac{(Yaa - Yab).Zba}{Yab}; \quad K2 = \frac{(Ybb - Yba).Zab}{Yba} \quad (\text{For any ratio})$$

Where, Zab and Zba are the proportionate ratio of A with B and B with A, respectively.

Therefore, product of Crowding Coefficient (K) = K1 × K2.

The values of K1 and K2 may be < = > 1 but value of K must be >1 for a biologically sustainable system. K =1 means there is no advantage from association and therefore, it is as good as one of the sole stand and if, K < 1 means there is a disadvantage from growing both species together.

5. Area Time Equivalent Ratio (ATER)

It is the per day yield received from the association as compared to their respective pure stands. The duration of intercrop due to long maturity of any one species may delay the harvesting of the association as compared to early harvest of any one of the species which may result in variation in per day productivity. It has significance where crop sequence or relay cropping is followed. In mono-cropped area it has not much importance since the plot remains fallow either it is harvested earlier or late.

Economical Parameters of Association

1. **Net-Returns:** Economical evaluation of any system is ultimately stronger than any other parameter of evaluation. Gross- returns of any enterprise does not sound much until and unless net-returns are not accounted. Therefore, significantly higher net-returns from the said association over sole stand is a must.

2. **Net-Returns/Re. Investment or Benefit: Cost Ratio:** Net-returns from an association may be higher but net-returns from each rupee of investment may not be higher. Therefore, this parameter may has an edge over in assessing the system only on the basis of net-returns.

3. Monetary Advantage (MA): It is another economical parameter based on biological parameter (LER) to assess the system.

MA (Rs.) =

Cost of crop A in mixed stand + cost of B in mixed stand $\times \dfrac{\text{LER} - 1}{\text{LER}}$

Monetary advantage must be positive and > 1. It will be positive if, LER of the association will be > 1 as well as higher the LER, higher will be the MA.

4. Relative Net-Return (RNR): It is the most accepted economical parameter for final conclusion of the results.

RNR (Rs.) =

$$\dfrac{\text{Cost of produce A in mind stand + cost of produce B in mixed stand} \pm (\text{Difference in cost of production of mixed stand and pure stand of A})}{\text{Cost of produce A in pure stand}}$$

The RNR in comparison to crop B can be also computed as above by substituting different in cost of production between mixed stand and pure stand of B and cost of produce B in pure stand.

The RNR from mixed stand vs. pure stand of at least A or B should be more than 1.

Based on the above proposed parameters, some of the experiments which were conducted in different parts of the world involving forage crops are summarized as under.

II. Forage Crops Sequences

Forage: Forage Systems: Mixed or intercrop stands of grass-legume or cereal: legume associations under different Agro-climatic conditions have been evaluated and recommended.

In round the year forage production system, in acidic alfisols of eastern India, intercropping of cowpea (*Vigna unguiculata*) between 1m row spacing of Hybrid Napier in *Kharif* season and berseem (*Trifolium alexandrinum*) in *rabi* season produced the maximum green herbage and was also accounted for the maximum monetary return (Prasad *et. al*, 1992) while cross sowing of sorghum (*Sorghum bicolor*) with cowpea with full seed rates of both the component species was suggested (Singh *et. al*, 1989). Intercropping of Teosinte (*Euclena maxicana*) with Ricebean in 2 : 1 row ratio significantly recorded the maximum forage yield and net profit. It has also saved the N application to 25% and maintained the initial soil N status (Choubey *et.al*, 1999).

Cross sowing of annual Deenanath grass (*Pennisetum pedicellatum*) and cowpea with full seed rates of both was found good for the maximum harvest of green and dry matter yields which computed for the maximum LER (1.52) as well as received the highest monetary advantage (Prasad *et. al*, 1990).

Intercropping of some perennial tropical grasses and legumes indicated that association of Palasid grass (*Bracharia brizantha*) with ricebean (*Phaseolus calcaratus*) in 1: 1 row ratio produced the highest herbage field as well as it gave the maximum net-returns while Thin Napier in 1:1 row ratio with Brazilian Lucerne (*Stylosanthes guianensis*) also gave a rich harvest fed with 4o kg/ha of both nitrogen and phosphorus (Prasad, 1981).

Mixed association of the three major Rabi season (temperate) forage crops; oats (*Avena sativa*), berseem/Egyptian clover (*Trifolium alexandrinum*) and lucerne (*Medicago sativa*) of northern India in paired rows can be feasible to harvest more nutritious forages.

Intercropping of oats with Chinese cabbage (*Brassica chinensis*) in 2: 1 row ratio or, broadcasting of Chinese cabbage seeds in oats rows with full seed rates of both the component species gave 20% more yield as well as 21% more net-returns over pure stand of oats (Prasad and Singh, 1991)

Under east African rain-fed conditions, Taye *et. al* (2007) recorded improvement in nutritive value of Napier grass mixed with either *Desmodium intortum* or *Lablab purpureus* at different stages of cutting of Napier grass while under the same agroclimatic conditions, Berhanu *et. al* (2007) advised for the cultivation of oats (*A. sativa*) and vetch (*Vicia villosa*) by keeping a seed mixture of 25% and 75% , respectively. It also computed for 32% advantage in yield (LER= 1.32).

Intercropping of *Cenchrus setigerus* and *Vigna unguiculata* in 1:2 row ratio in semi-arid conditions of Rajasthan with 40 kg N+ 24kg P/ha gave the highest yield of forages and CP and the same also accounted as the most remunerative pattern (Meena *et al.*, 2008).

Forage-Food crop systems

Growing of food and forage crops on the same unit of land can meet the demands of both the farmers as well as their livestock.

Introduction of either a forage or food legume with cereal or vice-versa can be biologically a better system. As such, sowing of 2 rows of Deenanath grass (*Pennisetum pedicellatum*) within 1m row space of Arhar (*Cajanus cajan*) can produce equally good quantity of forage to pure stand of grass along with 75% pulses to its sole seeding.

Wheat and Lucerne were also grown simultaneously in same unit of land successfully. Intercrop association of wheat at 80 cm row spacing and 3 rows of Lucerne at 20 cm apart within 2 rows of wheat can be done

Chapter 15

Nutrient Management

I. Essential Nutrients for Plants: Criterion for Essentiality of Nutrients

Arnon and Stout (1939) led down the 3 criteria for the essentiality of nutrients for plants. It states that

1. In absence of an element, it is not possible for plant to complete its life vegetative or reproductive cycle (life cycle)

2. The role played by an element is specific and it can not be replaced by any other element.

3. The element is directly involved in nutrition of the plant Deficiency of a nutrient is specific and substitution can not be done.

Accordingly, 16 nutrient elements are found as essential for the plants. Some scientists claim for 17 (Co) while some others for 19 (Ni and Si). These 16 elements are classified in to 2 groups.

Essential Nutrient elements				
Major / Macro-nutrients (> 1000 ppm)			Minor/ Micro-nutrients/ Trace elements (<50 ppm)	
Primary nutrients		Secondary nutrients		
C	N	Ca	Fe	Mn
H	P	Mg	Cu	B
O	K	S	Zn	Mo/Co, Cl

Table 15.1: Average Concentration of Mineral Nutrients in Plant Shoot Dry Matter (DM), Sufficient for Adquate Growth

Element	Available Form	Mmole/gDM	Mg/kg(ppm)	%	Relative At. No.
Mo	MoO_4^{--}	0.001	0.1	-	1
Cu	Cu^{++}	0.10	6	-	100
Zn	Zn^{++}	0.30	20	-	300
Mn	Mn^{++}	1.0	50	-	1000
Fe	Fe^{++}	2.0	100	-	2000
B	H3BO3$^-$	2.0	20	-	2000
Cl	Cl^-	3.0	100	-	3000
S	SO_4^{--}	30	-	0.1	30 000
P	$H_2PO_4^- : HPO_4^-$	60	-	0.2	60 000
Mg	Mg^{++}	80	-	0.2	80 000
Ca	Ca^{++}	125	-	0.5	125 000
K	K^+	250	-	1.0	250 000
N	NO_3^-, NH_4^+	1000	-	1.5	1 000 000

C, H and O constitute from 94-96% of plant body on dry weight basis, of which C and O each share 45% while H constitutes from 4-6% (Table 15.3). Thus, rest constitute from 4-6%. Air is the source of C and O is available from both water and air while H is taken only from water. The sources of N are from soils, fertilizers as well as atmosphere while rest from soils and mineral matters. The vertical rows also indicate the essentiality order as such, C is more essential to H and H is more essential to O. The same is also true for other rows. Since, the requirement of Fe in some plant species may be as higher as to some macronutrients hence it jumps to secondary nutrient group. Therefore, it is also known as border element. The requirement of Mo for some plant species may be as low as 1 ppb hence it is also known as ultra element. As the roles of Mo and Co are at least same in legumes thus, it acts as a substitute for Mo. Concentration of Cl in different sources of water is very high hence, its deficiency hardly occurs.

There 18 nutrients are essential for animals. Out of above 16 nutrients, B is neither an essential nutrient for animal nor human being. Therefore, 15 plus Na, I and Co are essential for animals and 18 plus florin ie, 19 nutrients are essential for human being.

II. Nutrients Concentration in Soils

On the basis of concentration of nutrients in soils, it is categorized into low, medium and high as presented in the Table 15.4.

Table 15.2: Nutrients in Soils and their Fertility Range

Nutrient	Unit	Fertility status		
		Low	Medium	High
Organic Carbon	(%)	< 0.50	0.50-0.75	> 0.75
Available Nitrogen	Kg/ha	< 280	280-560	> 560
Available Phosphorous	Kg/ha	< 20	20-40	> 40
Available Potash	Kg/ha	< 125	125-250	> 250
Available Sulphur	Kg/ha	< 20	20-30	>30
Available Boron	ppm	< 0.5	0.5-0.75	> 0.75
Available Zinc	ppm	< 0.60	0.6-1.2	> 1.2
Available Copper	ppm	< 0.20	0.2-0.4	>0.4
Avaible Iron	ppm	< 4.50	4.5-9.0	> 9.0
Available manganese	ppm	< 2.00	2.0-4.0	> 4.0
Available Molybdenum	ppm	< 0.05	0.05-0.10	> 0.10

Thus from the above table, we can estimate the approximate ratio of different nutrients. Among the macronutrients it is in the ratio of 1: 1: 8 :16 for S : P : K :N and for micronutrients it is in 1 :4 : 10 : 40 :90 for Mo : Cu : B/Zn : Mn : Fe, respectively.

III. Optimization of Nutrient in Forages

Nutrient optimization is more accountable in a present day cropping system since, in a soil-plant-animal/ human chain, deficiency of a particular nutrient in a soil system will lead to deficiency in plant species either it is a food crop or forage crop which is further transferred to human body resulting in to susceptibility of several diseases. Such phenomenon as a mall nutrition is more prevalent in developing countries. The optimization of a particular nutrient in plant species is done by testing the status of the nutrient in question either in soil or plant or in both.

1. Plant growth/ yield in relation to nutrient supply through soil: The optimum level of nutrient is applied either conducting the experiment in field or in glass house. The different levels of the said nutrient element are applied in replicated form. The growth of the plant or dry matter yield is taken to calibrate against the supplied levels of nutrient and is compared with the yield taken in presence of the optimum level of all nutrients versus yield under deficient level of a particular nutrient. This gives the reduction in yield under deficient conditions of the said nutrient. It also highlights the contribution of one nutrient element to yield (Fig.15.1).

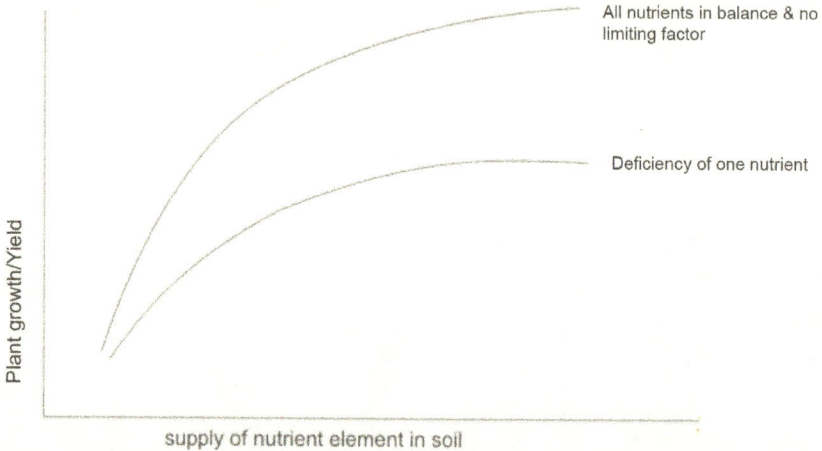

Fig. 15.1. Yield response to supply of nutrient in soil

Plant sample of the entire plant parts or fully expanded leaves just below the bud are taken for analysis of nutrient concentration and is correlated with the yields.

Optimum concentration of nutrient is that level of nutrient at which it is just sufficient or just deficient for the maximum growth/yield, while critical concentration of the nutrient is that at which 5 or 10 % reduction in optimum level of nutrient occurs (Ulrich and Hills, 1967)

2. Optimization of nutrient level based on plant diagnosis: The concentration of nutrient in plant samples grown at different levels of the same in soil is analyzed and plotted against the plant growth/ yields.

The graph (Fig. 15.2) representing the different zones indicates the relation between performance of plant growth/yield in presence of different concentrations of nutrient.

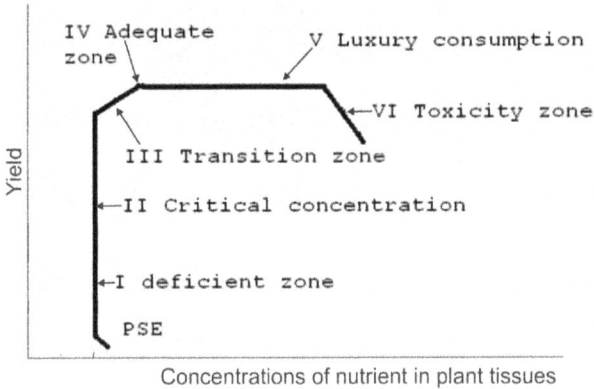

Fig.15. 2: Concentration of nutrient in plant and growth/yields.

I. **Deficient Zone:** Where > 80% reduction in yield is expected (Loneragan,1978)

II. **Critical Zone:** Where > 20 % reduction in yield is expected (Ulrich, 1972)

III. **Transition Zone:** Where 10 % reduction in yield is expected

IV. **Adequate Zone:** Where 100 % yield is expected and further increase in concentration of nutrient, the increase in yield is not expected and it is known as luxury consumption.

V. **Toxic Zone:** Where further increase in concentration of nutrient may reduce the growth/yield due to toxicity of the element.

Piper and Steenberg Effect (PSE) In wheat, Loneragan (1978) observed that Cu is readily lost from ageing leaves grown with adequate Cu concentration but it did not happen in plant deficient in Cu. This loss of Cu from sufficient Cu containing leaves was faster than that of Cu deficient leaves, is termed as Piper and Steenberg Effect.

This states that a plant grown under sufficient concentration of a nutrient may show deficiency very readily if, put under deficient conditions as compared to that already grown under in-adequate conditions.

On the basis of such observations, the critical concentrations of some of the forage species are listed as under

IV. Nutrients in Forages

Critical Concentration of Nutrient elements in some Forage Grasses and Legumes (CSIRO, Australia, Technical Bulletin, 1977) is presented in the Table 15.3.

Table 15.3: Nutrients in Forages

S. No.	Common and Scientific Names	Macro-nutrients (%)	Micro-nutrients (ppm)
A. Grasses			
1	Buffel / Anjan grass (*Cenchrus ciliaris*)	P- 0.12 S- 0.25	NA*
2	Columbus grass (*Sorghum almum*)	P- 0.20	NA
3	Guinea grass (*Panicum maximum*)	P-0.20 S- 0.12	NA
4	Kikuyu grass (*Pennisetum clandestinum*)	P- 0.22 S – 0.12	NA
5	Pangola grass (*Digitaria decumbens*)	P – 0.18 S – 0.12	NA
6	Paspalum (*Paspalum dialatum*)	P – 0.25 S – 0.12	0.25 0.12
7	Phalaris (*Phalaris aquatica*)	P – 0.25, K- 1.5 S- 0.2, Ca -0.25, Mg- 0.4	Cu - 40 and Zn -15
8	Rhodes grass (*Chloris gayana*)	NA	Mn -60, B - 5 and Mo - 0.3
9	*Perennial Rye grass (Lolium perenne)*	P – 0.35, K – 2.0, S – 0.27, Ca – 0.25 and Mg – 0. 16	Cu - 6,0, Zn - 14, Mn - 50, Fe - 50, B - 5 and Mo - 0.3
10	*Setaria (Setaria sphacelata)*	P – 0.21, K – 1.8 and S -0.12	NA
B. Legumes			
1	*Centro (Centrosema pubescens)*	P- 0.16 K-0.75	Cu - 5.0, Zn 20.0
2	Egyptian Clover (*Trifolium alexandrinum*)	P- 0.20, K – 0.70	Cu – 5.0
3	Kenya White Clover (*T. semipilosum*)	S – 0.17	NA
4	Strawberry Clover *(T. fragiferum)*	K – 1.0	Cu – 4.0
5	Subterranean Clover *(T. subterranean)*	P - 0.12, K -1.5, S – 0.25	Cu -4.0, Zn, 12.0, Mo - 0.15
6	White Clover (*T. repens*)	P – 0.25, K -1.1, S -0.20, Ca -1.0, Mg – 0.18 Cu, Zn, Mn Fe, B & Mo	0.25, 1.1 0.20, 1.0 & 0.18 % Cu -5.0, Zn - 15, Mn - 25, Fe - 50, B – 25, Mo - 0.15

Contd...

Contd...

S. No.	Common and Scientific Names	Macro-nutrients (%)	Micro-nutrients (ppm)
7	Glycine (*Neonotonia wightii*)	P – 0.23, K -0.8, S -0.17	Zn -22.0
8	Lucerne *(Medicago sativa)*	P – 0.25, K – 0.65, S -0.2, Ca -0.5, Mg – 0.31	Cu -10, Zn - 16, MN - 30, B - 35 Mo - 0.5
9	Phasey Bean (M*acroptilium lathyroides*)	P – 0.20, K - 0.75, S -0.15	NA
10	Siratro (*M. atropurpureum*)	P – 0.30, K – 0.75, S -0.20	Zn – 24
11	Brazilian Lucerne *(Stylosanthes guianensis)*	P -0.16, K 1.0, ca -1.5	NA
12	Shrub stylo *(S. capitata)*	P -0.11, K -1.0, Ca - 0.70	NA
13	River Hunter Lucerne (*S. hamata*)	P -0.13, K -1.0, Ca – 0.70	NA
14	S. Townsville (*S. humilis*)	P -0.17, K 0.6,Ca -0.7, S - 0.14	Zn - 34ppm
15	*S. macrophala*	P -0.10,K 0.9, Ca -0.8	NA

*NA- Not available

N concentrations on dry weight basis in grasses and cereals usually vary from 1.0 to 1.5 to a maximum of 2.0 per cent while in legumes from 2.0 to 3.5 per cent.

The Nitrogen Cycle

The nitrogen cycle has been given (Fig.15.3) below is self explanatory which is the combination of two cycles, one is the soil-plant-soil cycle in which the soil receives the nitrogen through animal and plant while the other involves in the loss of gaseous nitrogen to the atmosphere. A part of the latter is fixed by the N-fixing plants.

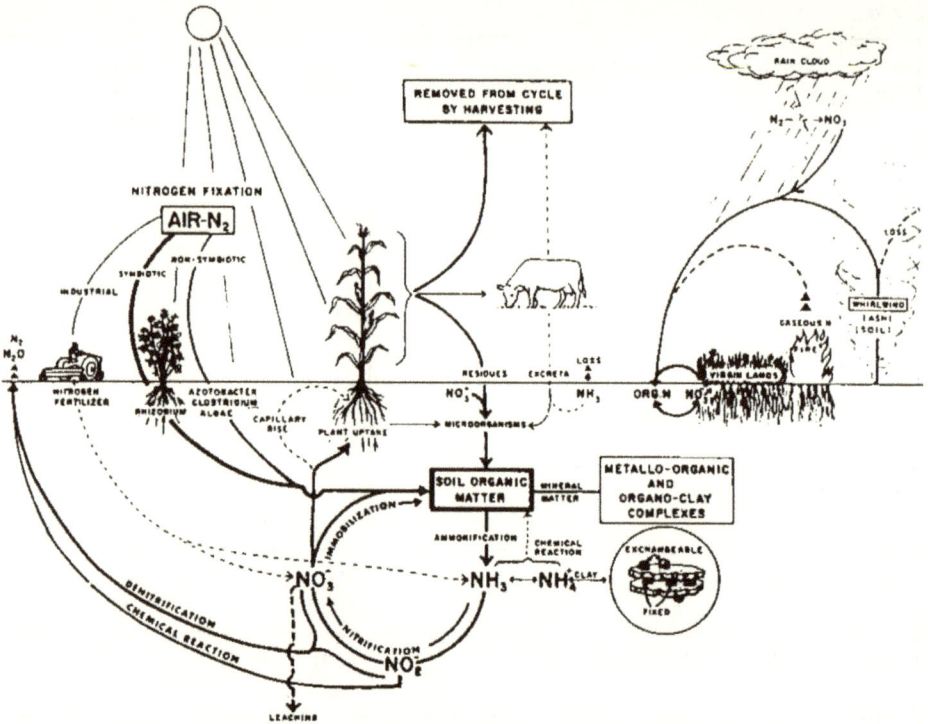

Fig.15.3. Schematic outline of nitrogen cycle

V. Some Facts in Forage Nutrition

1. Cation-Exchange-Capacity (CES) and Nutrient absorption

The root CEC to per unit root surface area of pulses crops is double to cereals and grasses. Ingeneal, the root CEC to per unit root surface area of forage legumes is double to food legumes hence, root CEC of forage legumes is 4 times to cereals but the total root CEC of grasses is higher to legumes due to higher root bio-mass resulting also in higher root surface area. Among the different legumes, lucerne has the highest CEC to per unit root surface area. Since species having high root CEC are more efficient in nutrients absorption together with higher affinity for strong cations usually under unfavourable conditions of soil, nutrients, moisture and temperature. As such, under moisture stress conditions in acid soils where availability of P, Ca and B is inadequate, dominancy of strong cations as well as affinity of Lucerne for these cations, restrict the adsorption of weaker cations in general and anions in particular which is unfavourable for growth of legumes. Though, the essentiality of weaker cations and anions is more to legumes but affinity is for strong cations, is a negative point for lucerne production under adverse conditions.

2. Phosphorus Requirement of Grasses and Legumes

The P requirement of legumes is higher than grasses and cereals which are not due to higher extraction from soils but due to higher Thresh Hold Value (THV) or critical concentration of legumes. Since, the grasses and cereals give higher yield hence, total harvest of P is also higher as compared to legumes, even a little higher concentration of P in legumes failed to extract more P than non-legumes due to low yield. It means that legume growing soils remained richer in soil-P after the harvest of the crop. Therefore, as per net P harvest efficiency, the P requirement of legumes is low as compared to cereals and grasses.

3. P availability in acid soils

The P availability and extraction by different crops in acid soils is the lowest (9-10%) as copared to any other soils (Sekhon and Puri, 1986). Even application of lime in acid soils does not facilitate in releasing of already fixed or previously applied P. Even a decrease in availability of previously added P at all levels of lime was recorded.The crop response to liming was recorded not due to P availability but it due to the effect of Ca, supplied through lime and release of P through decomposition of organic matter(Soltanpour *et al.*, 1974).

4. Top-dressing of Nitrogen in standing legumes

The N requirement of legumes is less than grasses and cereals due to ability to fix atmospheric N. A small quantity of N as a basal dose is only applied as a source to nourish the young seedlings since topdressing of N in standing legumes in general and in amid or ammoniac forms is not recommended. This is due to the fact that the concentration of oxygen in soils in general and in moist soils is limited. Since the amide or ammonical forms of nitrogen requires oxygen for nitrification and at the same time nodules bacteria also require oxygen for their multiplication hence, a competition for oxygen starts in which chemical source of nitrogen dominate in utilization of soils oxygen and as a result, the bacteria are devoid of oxygen die. Bishop *et al.* (1976) demonstrated 65% reduction of nitrogenase activity in 4 days in soybean in presence of 5mM $(NH_4)_2SO_4$ while Houward (1978) recorded inhibiting effects of NH_4^+ by a deviation in ATP supply. Therefore, such crop needs regular application of nitrogen if, once applied since there is an inadequate fixation of nitrogen in absence of proper population of bacteria. Hence, such practice is neither scincitific nor economical.

5. Folliar Application of Nutrients

In plant system, the uptake of nutrients takes place through xylem vessels but translocation of some of the nutrients occurs through both xylem and phloem while some to them have only phloem transport. On the basis of transport of mineral nutrients in plant roots studied by Marschner and Richter (1973) and other workers, it can be concluded that since, the transport of N occurs both in upward and lower directions through xylem and phloem, hence, soil as well as foliar application of N is suggested but as the P is not translocated through phloem hence, foliar application of P fertilizers is not suggested. K^+ and Na^+ are transported in both directions but phloem-immobile Ca^+ ion is exclusively moves upward to the shoot while water moves downward to the root. Thus, movement of Ca^{++} and water is antagonistic to each other. Similarly, since B is not taken up by the phloem hence spray application of this nutrient is not suggested. In case of B deficiency in cauliflower, spray application is only effective in flower to some extent however, the die-heart or hollowness of the stem remains as such. Therefore, the soil application of B is preferred.

6. Conditions for Maximum Availability of Nutrients

The N nutrition is dependent on C: N ratio in the soils. The C: N ratio from 12: 1 to 15: 1 is ideal for equilibrium for mineralization and immobilization of N which results in to optimum availability of the same. Ratio below 12:1 increases the mineralization and loss of N while ratio above 15:1 increases the immobilization and reduces the availability of N. Besides, this soil moisture and temperature are also accountable for nutralization of nutrients. Soil moisture just above Field Capacity (FC) is favourable for N availability. Soil temperature between 30-40°C is good for tropical legumes for higher N-fixatation where as for temperate legumes it should be 15 – 25°C. Since, N and S have synergestic relation hence, N: S ratio of 10: 1 to 16: 1 is said to be ideal for their nutrition but in some cases, ratio below and above may show deficiency of the either elements.

The P nutrition to plants is entirely dependent on soil pH. At pH 6.5, since the ratio of $H_2PO_4^-$ and HPO_4^{--} remains at 50 : 50 hence, it results in to maximum availability of this nutrient. At low pH, increase in $H_2PO_4^-$ and at high pH increase in HPO_4^{-2} or even $PO4^{-3}$ ions charges this ratio, results in low availability of phosphorous.

Though, The nutrition of K is not directly affected by C : N ratio and soil pH however, high concentration of Al ions at low pH restricts the K to adsorb at the root surfaces. Application of lime in acid soils with replacement of Al by Ca from the absorption site, becomes relatively easier for K to replace the di-valent (Ca) as compared to tri-valent (Al).

It is also to note down that about 70-75 % of externally applied N, P, K in the soils is lost through leaching, volatilization, leacing, runoff, fixation and several other process. Thus, only 25-30 % of nutrients which is taken by the plant, is further lost to the extent of 70-75% of total uptake (25-30%) in different physiological processes.

7. Biological Nitrogen Fixatation

The "nef" gene is responsible for bio-logical fixatation by plants.

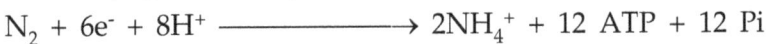

$$N_2 + 6e^- + 8H^+ \longrightarrow 2NH_4^+ + 12\ ATP + 12\ Pi$$

$$\text{nef}$$
$$2H^+ + 2\ e^- + 4ATP \longrightarrow H_2 + 4ADP = 4Pi$$

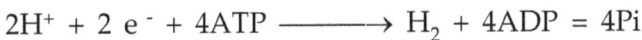

The overall reactions given above are catalized by the nitrogenase in bacteroides nodules in presence of the 'nef' gene. The presence of leghemoglobin in the nodules act as O_2 carrier in the same way as to that of blood hemoglobin Different plant species are capable to fix the nitrogen with different capacity. As such *Leucaena leuclaocepha* fixes the highest quantity of N (560 kg N/ha/yr) followed by *Centrosema pubescens* (280 kg N/ha/yr), *Medicago sativa* (150 kgN/ha/yr) and others. Among different legumes, Lucerne usually transfers about 40-45 % of self fixed-N to associated grasses while only 10 % of self fixed-N is transferred by *Stylosanthes guinensis* to its companion grasses or say, itself utilizes 90 % of N that is why, being a legume, it dominates over grasses in association.

8. Plant Resistant to Nutrient Deficiency and Toxicity

The P requirement of legumes is usually higher than grasses and cereals but its requirement for some of the pasture legumes are even less than many grasses and cereals. The critical concentration of soil-P for *Stylosanthes species* in general and of *S. guianensis* is as low as 2.5 ppm, is just equal to the need of *Andropogon gayanus*.

The toxicity of elements like Al and Fe is more prevalent in acid soils in which major area of pasture is managed through out the world. The plant species may perform well in these soils due to either its requirement for the said toxic nutrient say, Fe may be high or it may restrict the absorption of such elements through chelating (claw catching) or making complex ions with the organic acids released by the roots (Hoffland, 1992). On the basis of nutrients concentrations in different forage grass and legumes species obserbed by Mishra (2002), it can be enterpreted that even rice straw produced in high iron containing acid soils contains very high concentration of Fe (>400ppm) to those grown in neutral or slightly high pH soils (246ppm) but several forage species viz. Thine Napier grass, *Brachiaria* species, Guinea grass, *Andropogon* species and *Leucaena* even grown in acid soils cotain very low concentration of Fe (104-128ppm). This might be due to the fact that the roots of some of the plant species secret some organic acids which form complex ions with the toxic elements (Al and Fe). Since, the size of complex ions is larger than the original ions, hence their entry into the xylem vessels is restricted and plant grows well even under toxic level of the said elements. Some times external application of chelating agents is also done to complex these ions to restrict their toxicity.

In other case, if the requirement of some plant species for the said elements is itself high then such species may sustain well even under toxic conditions of those elements. Such as forage crops like *Cassia* species (282 ppm Fe), *Stylosanthes* species (272 ppm Fe) and Hybrid Napier (171ppm Fe) grown well in high Fe containing soils due to their higher requirement for the nutrient in question.

Chapter 16
Agroforestry

History

The importance of trees in civilization is nothing but the synchronization of the both. As such, the records of *Kalpvriksh* in *Bhagawat Puran* it self speakes its significance which means that the survival of trees are must since they are supporting and regulating the life of entire organisms through their different products.

Agnipuran of 1,000 BC further highlighted the plantation of trees as a noble act. It says that 10 wells are equal to one tank, 10 tanks are equal to one lake, 10 lakes are equal to one son and 10 sons are equal to one tree for earning blessing due to the fact that plant is the only source of trapping solar energy for man kind. It is also said where ever man goes, pollution goes together and only plant clears the pollution. Lord *Buddha* before 2500 years also identified the importance of *Bodhi* tree to become Lord. Description of Dandakaraniya in *Ramayan* and *Pipal* tree in Holy *Gita* where Lord Krishna declared himself as " Among the trees, I am the *Pipal* tree".

The shifting cultivation resulted in deforestation and changes in ecological system hence growing of trees and field and forage crops simultaneously in association gave birth to the term "Agroforestry'. In India and elsewhere, research on Agroforestry came into existence at IGFRI, Jhansi, CSWCR and TI, Dehradun, CAZRI, Jodhpur and ICAR Complex for NE Hill Region during 1962 to 1970.

The National Commission on Agriculture introduced the syllabus on Agroforestry in all the SAUs during seventh five-year plan period. Presently, about 40 Agroforestry centres are working in the country and some of the Universities have also started Post Graduate programme in this field.

Definitions

As early as Bene *et al.* (1977) defined the Agroforestry as a sustainable management system for land that increases overall production, combines agricultural crops, trees/forest plants and/or animals simultaneously or subsequently and applies management practices that are compatible with cultural patterns of local population.

Just in the succeeding year, King and Chandler (1978) stated that Agroforestry is a sustainable land management system which increases the overall yield of land, combines the production of crops and forest plants and/or animal simultaneously or subsequently on the same unit of land and applies management practices that are compatible with cultural pattern of local population. Nair (1979) also defined the Agroforestry as a land use system that integrates trees, crops and animals in a way that is scientifically sound, economically desirable, practically feasible and socially acceptable to the farmers.

In 1982, Lundegren also defined the Agroforestry as a collective term for land use systems of woody perennials (shrubs and trees) are grown in association with crops and pasture (herbs) and/or livestock in a spatial arrangement, a rotation or both to keep both ecological and economical interactions between these species.

Thus, all these definitions are not more than definitions of inter/ mixed cropping in which maximum exploitation of the natural resources on the same unit of land is taken or say, it is a combination of forest trees/horticulture trees+crops/forages + animals on the same unit of land.

Importance

Global demands for fuel energy, food, forages and timber are going to be a serious challenge in developing countries in near future. According to an estimate, fuel wood demand of 130 ml. tones in 1980 has presently increased to 158ml.tonnes. There is also demand for 27ml.m^3 of timber against the supply of only12 ml.m^3. The gap between demand and supply of fodder is also alarming since, we are only meeting 50%

requirement of our animals. Thus, pressure on our forest is mounting day by day which has shrinked to 22.5% of geographical area. The situation in other developing countries is more serious. In some of the African countries the shortage of fire wood is as serious as to food. As such only 2.5% of land is only covered in sub-Sahara region of East Africa where annually one ml.ha. forest lands are on degradation. Only 0.11 ha/capita forest cover is available in India as compared to 12, 70 and 130 ha in USA, Australia and Canada, respectively. Therefore, putting of non-culturable wastelands under Agroforestry system can be only way out to meet the present day challenges for fuel, forage and timber since, we can not spare crop lands due to equally demand for food.

Concept

The concept of growing trees along with crops is not a new concept in either developed or developing countries. However, the demographic compulsion for demand of food exerted enough pressure on tree vegetation and accordingly not only trees but even horticultural plants were also cut and cleaned for field crops. Therefore, plantation of trees atleast along the boundry of the lands besides road sides and rivers banks has resulted as National priority.

Principles

Mutually biological cohesiveness among the component species is a must for any Agroforestry system. Growing trees on degraded highlands and wastelands may further improve the soil conditions as well as micro-climate. Growing trees with crops in proper spatial arrangement and time without any reduction in yield can be a viable system. Even increases in total productivity to per unit land area may be an additional advantage.

Objectives

The main objectives of this biological system may be out lined as:

1. Higher biomass production as compared to sole stand to meet fuel, forage, food, fruits and timber demands from same unit of land.

2. Soil Fertility enhancement due to presence of N-fixing trees even presence of trees and grasses improved the soil physical conditions and conserve the top fertile soils from erosion.

3. Besides availability of food, forages, fuels etc. it also provides raw materials to small agro-industries for pulp, paper, fibre, gum, wax, essential oils, resin, lac, dye, tannins,and perfumes making.

4. It also helps in changing the micro-climate by lowering the temperature which is more felt during scorching sunlight in arid and semi-arid regions.

5. It may also generate employement to rural mass to some extent.

Scope

Swelling human and livestock population is a challenging task to meet their requirement for food, forage and fuel energy. The horizontal expansion of plant has a very little scope due to limited land resources. Therefore, vertical expansion is the only feasibility to meet our present and future requirement. Agroforestry of multistorage farming system is the only solution to harvest more and more solar energy in general and especially from waste and marginal lands.There is a need to identify the region based technology hence, the ICAR has already initiated AICRP on Agroforetry during 1983 and presently about 40 centres are working on this aspect.

Types -The Agroforestry system can be broadly classified into the following types.

A. Based on structure

1. Agri-silviculture system (Crops in the main land and trees on the boundry).

2. Silvi-pastual system (Improved pasture species with woody perennials).

3. Agri-silvi-pastural system (Combination of crops plus trees and pasture species with animal components which needs more precision).

4. Multipurpose Foretry system (Growing of forest as well as fruit trees for forage, fuel, flowers, fruits, resin, medicines, lac, silk and gum etc.

5. Silvi-pastural system (Managing trees and pasture species with suitable grazing system, best followed in arid and semi-arid conditions).

B. Based on major components: The nomenculture has been done starting with the dominant or major components and the purpose to which it is established.

1. Agro-silviculture (Crops are primary and trees are secondary components).
2. Silvi-agriculture (Trees are major and crops are minor components)
3. Pastural-silviculture (Pasture species are the major and trees are minor).
4. Silvo-pastural (Trees are major and pasture species are minor)
5. Silvo-agri-pasture (Dominated by trees and followed by crops and pasture).
6. Agro-silvi-pasural (Dominated by crops and followed by trees and pasture).

C. Based on allied enterprises

Besides the combinations of crops, pasture and trees/horticultural components, the system may enclude apiculture, sericulture, lac-culture and pisci-culture and thus, it may be desinated as Agroforestry-cum-apiculture/sericulture/lac-culture/pisiculture, accordingly.

Advantages

a. Increases total productivity of the land
b. Improves soil physical and chemical properties/fertility
c. Improves the micro-climate
d. Provides food, forages, timber, fuels and other different agro-industrial products
e. Increases employement and income for better socio-economic conditions.
f. Increases in conversion of non-culturable lands into culturable one.
g. Brings out improvement in problematic soils.

Chapter 17

Forages in Soil Conservation

Loss of soil and water through erosion is one of the biggest menance in crop production system. A very heavy quantity of soil (5,333 mt/year or 16.35 t/ha of soil is detaiched every year of that 29% is transported to sea by different rivers and 10% is deposited in the reservoirs. Beside this, 2.5 mtN, 3.3 mt P_2O_5 and 2.6 mt K_2O are lost away early. Deforestation, over grazing, shifting cultivation and cropping on unterraced undulating lands resulting drought in uplands and flooding of low lands.

Pasture and rangeland species due to their well developed root sustem as well as canopy structure are more efficient in binding the soil and giving an adequate cover to control the soil erosion. Forage grasses and legumes help the soils in the following ways by

- reducing the impact of rain drops on soil surface
- slowing down the velocity of run-off water
- binding the soil texture and improving the soil structure
- improving the water stable aggregates in soils
- increasing the soil water infiltration rate
- improving the soils physico-chemical properties and fertility
- reducing the velocity of water in water- ways of watersheds

The soil conserving capacity of different grass and legume species varies which is measured by termed as conservation value. Ambasht (1977) proposed an equation to estimate this value.

$$CV = 100 - \frac{SWP}{SWO} \times 100$$

Where,

CV is the conservation value in percentage

SWP is the weight of soil washed out from plant covered plot

SWO is the weight of soil washes out from bare plot

On this basis the soil conservation values for *Saccharum bengalensis* (95.5%0, *Cynodon dactylon* (94.4%) and *Ciperus rotendus* (92.9) were recorded.

The works done on these above aspects since 1956 and onwards for the period of about two decades at DVC Hazaribagh and Ranchi, Jharkhand, India indicated that

– Marvel grass (*Dicanthium annulatum*) was assessed as the best grass for high soil binding capacity under upland conditions.

– *Pennisetum purpureum, Panicum maximum, Pennisetum polystachyon* and *Chloris gayana* with their high root weight were more efficient in improving infiltration rate and stable aggregate.

– Soil organic matter and water stable aggregate were increased significantly under the cover of *P. polystachyon, P. pedecellatum, Andropogon gayanus* and *Braichiaria brizantha* grasses.

– The minimum soil loss was also recorded under the cover of *Cynodon plectostachyus, P. polystachyon* and *Urochloa stolonifera*.

– A better canopy was developed under the mixed stands of *Stylosanthes guinensis* with *P. pedecellatum* or *A. gayanus*.

A large number of trials were conducted at differen regions of India on the soil and water conserving efficiency of different grass and legume species indicated a significant contribution in their conserving efficiencies of these two vital inputs.

Soil and water loss under different grass covers on 0.5 and 1.0% slopes at Kota indicated that in 0.5% slope, *Dichanthium annulatum* binds the soil most effectively followed by *Cynodon dactylon*.The loss of nutrients (N, P, and K) was much higher under grain crops as compared to grass (Table 17.1).

Table 17.1 Soil, Water and Nutrient Losses at 1% Slope at Kota Clay Soil

Treatment	Water loss (mm)	Soil loss (mm)	N loss (kg/ha	P₂O₅ loss (kg/ha)	K₂O loss (Kg/ha)
Dichanthium annulatum	20	0.06	1.2	0.8	16.8
Cultivated fallow	175	8.90	11.1	8.3	69.3
Blackgram	138	5.40	8.7	5.5	570.8
Soybean	143	4.50	7.9	6.2	397.9
Cowpea	84	2.90	7.3	3.4	331.1
Jowar+ Arhar	106	3.20	7.2	4.5	282.3

A very detailed study done by Chaterjee and Maiti (1974) on the role of grasses in soil conservation for continuous 15 years in Alfisols of Ranchi (East Inddia) indicated effectiveness of grasses in sand stabilization, developed roots and improvement in water-stable aggregates and pore spaces of soil, reduced run-off and soil loss and build up the soil fertility (Table 17.2). They suggested that good soils with 1 to 2% slopes should be put under crops while grasses on steeper slopes are good for crop production.

Table 17.2: Run-off and Soil loss under Different Systems of Land Use in Ranchi (India)

Grass	Run off (%)	Soil loss (kg/ha)
Cynodon Dactylon	35	56
Cenchrus ciliaris	33	134
Panicum antidotale	36	403
Pennisetum Polystachyon	27	67
Urochloa stolonifera	32	78
Grassland management		
Over grazed	27	2,352
Properly grazed	19	785
Not grazed	11	392
Land use		
Untouched fallow	11	583
Properly grazed fallow	22	857
Overgrazed fallow	22	3,280
Upland rice (direct seeded)	14	2,792
Maize cropping	6	3,276

Hadimani *et. al.* (1972) at Dharwar recorded *Pennisetum clandestinum, Tripogon bromoides, Eragrosts amabilis* and *Cynodon dactylon* as superior soils binders.while *Themeda triandra, Ischaemum indicum* and *paspalum dilatatum* are for good soil stabilizers. The herb *Centella asiatica* though developing a flat and dense canopy has not proved an efficient soil binder in consonance with good surface cover produced.

At Dehradun runoff and soil loss on 9 per cent slop under grass cover (*Cynodon dactylon*) was just 2.1 t/ha as compared to 15056.0 t/ha under bare fallow during June-October having 1250 mm rainfall. Even natural grass cover was more efficient in controlling the soils which allowed only 1.0 t/ha of soil loss and no loss of soil during November- March under 173 mm rainfall (Table 17.3).

Table 17.3 Runoff and Soil loss on 9% Slop in Dehradoon during Monsoon and Dry

Treatment	June-October (RF 1250mm), Soil loss (t/ha)	November-March (RF 173mm) Soil loss (t/ha)
Grass cover (*Cynodon*)	2.1	0.2
Bare fallow	42.4	3.6
Bare ploughed	156.0	5.8
Natural grass	1.0	0.0

Role of grasses in conserving the soil under high rainfall conditions (1250mm) conditions of Rajasthan also indicated only 2.1 t/ha/year of soil loss while maize cover allowed a loss of 28.5 t soil/ha/year. However cowpea was even more efficient in controlling the soil loss (1.3 t/ha/year) in comparision to grasses.

Under plateau conditions of Hyderabad (AP) *Dicanthium annulatum* allowed only a few kg of soil loss (0.06 t/ha/year) under1250mm of raionfall (Table17.4) while among crops, cowpea + safflower was more effective and cultivated fallow was the least.

Table 17.4: Soil Loss under Different Cropping Sequences in Hyderabad

Treatment	Soil loss (t/ha/yr) Rainfall (1250mm)
Jowar - Pigeonpea	3.19
Cowpea -Safflower	2.87
Soyabean - Safflower	4.46
Blackgram - Safflower	5.37
Dichanthium annulatum	0.06
Cultivated fallow	8.94

At high altitude (1500 mm) of Nilgiri hills in South India. role of one of the African grass Kikkuya grass (*Pennisetum cladestinum*) in conserving the soil was quite apparent along with producing the highest green herbage yield (7-9 t/ha). The other grass like *Eragrostis curuvulu* was also effective in controlling the soil loss. In watershed area of Tamil Nadu, Khas/Vetiver (*Veteveria zinanioides*) was found as the best barrier to control the soil loss, while in highly eroded conditions of Jharkhand plateau planting of lemon grass (*Cymbopogon ciotratus)* and other species was found as a better option to control gully erosion due in their developed root saystem and did not damage by the livestock due to non-palatable quality.

In Rajasthan, where in addition to soil loss through water, wind-erosion is a too serious problem, Planting of different grass species in different zones under different soil types and variable rainfall conditions is recommended (Table 17.5).

Table 17.5 : Grass Species for Different Regions of Rajasthan under different Rainfall

Soil type	ZoneA-200mm	ZoneB-300mm	ZoneC-400mm	ZoneD->400mm
Light soil	Aristida-Cenchrus	Lasiurus	Cenchrus	Dichanthium
Medium soil	Aristida-Eleusive	Sindicus	Cymbopogon	Cenchrus
Saline soil	Cenchrus-Sporobolus	Cenchrus	Dichanthium	Cenchrus
Rocky soil	Aristida-Eleusive	Cymbopogon	C.cetigerus	C.cetigerus

Role of grasses in Western Rangeland of America has also been evaluated by Aden (2007) who recommended use of shallow rooted grasses in place of deep rooted trees to increase water table in area receiving more than 450 mm of rainfall. Planting of grasses resulted in stream reaches with different patterns of river bank stability, erosion channels morphology, hydrology, increases in organic matter and trapping suspended sediments (John Lyons, *et al.*, 2007) while Gutirraz and Hernandez (1996) also recorded several benefits like decreases in runoff and internal erosion and improvement in soil organic matter by both above and under ground growth in seeding of grasses in semi-arid rangeland of north Mexico.

Therefore, it is an established fact that use of forage and other grasses as well as legumes as animal feed, their role in stablising soils and retaining soil water and fertility are equally compatable in farming system.

References

Aden R Hibbert.2007. Water yield improvement potential by vegetation management on Western Rangeland. *Jawara J. Am. Water Resource Association.* **19** (3) 375-381.

Ambast, R S.1971. Conservation of soil through plant cover on certain alluvial slopes in India IUCN/11 T. M. A. 4.

Arnon D L and Stout P R.1939. The essentiality of certain Elements in minute quality for Plants with Special Reference to Copper. *Plant Physiology.* **14:** 371-75.

Bene JG, Beall HW and Cote A. 1977. Trees, Food and People IDRC, Ottawa, Canada.

Berhanu A, Solomon M and Prasad N K. 2007. Effects of varying seed proportions and harvesting stages on biological compatibility and forage yield of oats (*A. sativa*) and vetch (*Vicia villosa* R) mixtures. *Livestock Research for Rural Devlopment* **19** (1): 1-13.

Bhagat R K, Prasad, N K and Singh A P. 1985. Response of boron and Molybdenum on forage production of Lucerne under limed and un-limed conditions. *Indian J. Agronomy* **(30)**: 332-41.

Bhagat R K, Prasad, N K and Singh A P. 1992. Nitrogen level and spacing of Hybrid Napier intercropped with legemes. J. of Res. (BAU) **4**(1): 67-69.

Bishop Pe, Guevera JG, Engelke, Evans HJ. 1976. Relation between glutamine synthetase and nitrogenase activities in the symbiotic association between *Rhizobium japonicum* and *Glycine max. Plant Physiol* **57:** 542-546

Boruah A R and Mathur B P.1979. Effect of cutting management and N fertilization on growth, yield and of fodder oats. *Indian J. Agronomy* **24**:50-53.

Burton G W. 1944. Hybrid between Napier grass and cattail millet. *Journal of Heredity*.**15**: 226-32.

Burton G W. 1965. Pearl millet Tift 23 A released. *Crops and Soils*. **17**: 197-241.

Chatterjee, B N 1954. Deenanath grass a fodder crop for Bihar. *Indian Farming*. **3**:16-17

Chaterjee B N.1973. The Seminar on the Agri. Develop. in N E India.

Chatterjee, B N and Maithi S.1974. Role of grasses in soil conservation in eastern India. *Soil Conserv. Digest*. **2** (1): 15-23.

Choubey S, Bhagat R K, Srivastava V C and Prasad N K. 1999. Effect of planting pattern on teosentie: ricebean intercropping. *Indian* J. of *Agronomy* **44**:525-29.

Cole, M M. 1963. Vegetation nomenclature and Classification with particular reference to the savanna, *So. Afr. Geo. J.* **45**: 3-4.

Dabadghao P M and Shankarnarayan K A. 1973. The grass cover of India. ICAR, New Delhi. 713 pp.

Epstein E. 1965. Mineral metabolism. In 'Plant Biochemistry' (J. Boner and J. E. Varner,eds.). pp. 438-66 Academic Press, London.

Gupta, V P.1974. Inter and intra-specific hybridization in forage plants – genus *Pennisetum*. *Indian J. of Genetics and Plant Breeding* **34A**,162-72.

Gutierraz, J and Hermandez . 1996. Runoff and interril erosion as affected by grass cover in a semi-arid rangeland of North Mexico. *J. of Arid Environments* **(34)** 3: 3287-295.

Hadimani, A S , Gumaste, S K, Joshi, V S and Patil S B. Effect of different grasses on aggregate stability and infiltration rates in red-sandy-clayloam soil. *J. of soil water conserv. India* **21**: 1-7.

Hatch M D and Slack C R. 1966. Photosynthesis by sugarcane leaves. A newcarboxylation reaction and the pathways of sugar formation. *Biochem. J*.**101**:103-11.

Heady H F. 1975. Rangeland Management, Mc Graw-hill:New York.

Hoffland E. 1992.Quantitative evaluation of the role of organic acid exudation in the mobilization of rock phosphate by rape. *Plant Soil* **140**:279-89.

Houward F. 1978. Influence of ammonium chloride on the nitrogenase activity of nodulated pea plant (*Pisum sativum*). *Appl Environm Microbiol* **35**: 1061-1065.

Hutton E M.1970. Tropical Pastures, *Adv. Agron.* **22**:1-23.

John Lyons, Stanley, W Thimble, Laura K Paine. 2007. Grasses vs trees Managing Riparian area to benifit stream of Central- North America. *J. of Am. Wte. Res. Association.* **38** (4): 910-930.

Josi Y P, Verma S S and Bhilare R L. 2007. Effect of Zinc levels on growth and yield of oat (*Avena sativa* L.) *Forage Research.* **32** (4): 238-39.

King K F S and Chandler L T. 1978. The Waste Lands ICARF, Nairobi, Kenya.

Kipps M S.1959. Production of Field Crops, Tata Mc Graw-Hill Publishing Co. Ltd. Bombay and New Delhi.

Krishnaswamy N and Raman V S. 1951. Cytogenetic studies in the interspecific hybrid of P. typhoides x P. *purpureum. Proc. of the First Scientific Workers Conference in AC and RI Coimbatore*, 47-71. (In PBA **26**:122).

Kumar P and Prasad N K. Biological and economical sustainability of forage maize (*Zea mays*) + cowpea (*V. unguiculata*) intercropping. *Indian J. of Agril. Sci.* **73**: 341-42.

Loneragan J F. 1978. Anomalis in the relationship of nutrient concentrations to plant yield. In: Fergusan A R, Bileski R L, Fergusan I B (eds.) Plant nutrition 1978. DSIR Inf. Ser. 134. Government Printer Wellington

Lundegren B O. 1982, Cited in editorial: What is Agroforestry? Agroforestry systems **1**:72.

Mannetje L. 't.1966. Stylosanthesis species, CSIRO, Division of Crops and Pasture. Ann. Report, p.45.

Marchner H, Richter C. 1973. Akkumulation translocation von K^+, Na^+ Ca= beiAngebot zu einzelnen Wurzelzonen von Maiskeimpflanzen. Z.Pflanzenernaechr. Bodenkd **235**:1-15.

Meena L R, Mann J S and Chand Roop 2008. Effect of intercropping row ratio and integrated nutrient management on the forage productivity and economic return from Dhaman grass (*Cenchrus setigerus* L) and cowpea (*Vigna unguiculata* L.) under semi-arid conditions. *Forage Research.* **33**(4): 219-23.

Mishra, S N (2002). Studies on micronutrients in soil, feeds, fodder, Rumen liquor and blood in cattle. Thesis submitted, Dept. of Vety. Medicine, BAU, Ranchi.

Mukherjee, A. K., Rana, S.K., Banerjee, S. Raquib, M.A. and Chaterjee, B.N.1981.Effect of fertilizer and row spacing on the yield of Dinanath grass. *Forage Res.* 7:97-99.

Nair P K R. 1979. Intensive Multiple Croping with Coconut in India: Princples, Progress and Prospects, Verlag Paual Paney, Berlin, Germany

Narwal, S.S., Tomar, P.S. and Paroda, A.S.1977. Effect of nitrogen and phosphorus levels with varying seed rates on fodder yield and quality of Deenanath grass. *Forage Res.*3:61-67.

Prasad, N K. 1981. Effect on production of grasses on the yield of Schofield Stylo on P levels. Indian *J. of Agronomy* **26**: 349-50

Prasad L K, Rahman A and Prasad N K. 1982. Effect of Cutting management intervals and N levels on herbage growth and yield of grasses. Indian *J. of Agronomy.* **27**: 103-06

Prasad L K, Rahman A and Prasad, N K. 1981. Evaluation of some pasture grasses to N levels. *Proc. Bihar Acad. Agril. Sci.* **(28)**: 63-64

Prasad N K, R K Bhagat and A P Singh.1988. Effect of cutting management, rate and time of seed production of Lucerne. *Indian J. Agronomy* **33**: 356-58.

Prasad N K, Bhagat R K and Singh A P. 1990. Intercropping of Deenanath grass *(P. pedicellatum)* with cowpea *(V. unguiculata)* for forage production. *Indian J. Agril. Sci.* **60**:15-18.

Prasad N K and Kumar P. 1995. Prasad, N K and Kumar, P. 1995, Evaluation of hybrid Napier *(P. purpureum)* genotypes under different levels of N for forage production in rain-fed conditions. *Indian J. of Agronomy* **(40)**: 164-65.

Prasad N K and Prasad L K. 1977. Evaluation of grasses under seepage conditions of Chotanagpur Plateau. *Indian J. of Agronomy* **(22)**: 183-85

Prasad N K and Singh A P. 1989. Forage yield of sorghum with legume. *Bihar Acad.of Agril. Sci.* **38**: 25-27.

Prasad N K and Singh A P. 1989. Wheat: Lucerne intercropping associations. National Symp. Strategy for forage production and improvement by 2000 AD. *Special Bulletin* IGFRI. 1884.

Prasad N K and Singh A P. 1991. Biological potential and economic feasibility of Wheat: Lucerne intercropping system. *Indian J. of Agril. Sci.* **61**: 838-40.

Prasad N K and Singh A P. 1991. Biological potential and economic feasibility of oats (*A. sativa*) and Chinese cabbage (*B. chinensis*) intercropping system for forage production. *Indian J. of Agronomy*.36: 71-77.

Prasad N K and Singh A P. 1992. Influence of P carriers and levels of lime on forage production of Egyptian clover (*T. alexandrinum*) and Lucerne (*M. sativa*) and their residual effect on Deenanath grass *(P. pedicellatum)*. *Indian J. of Agronomy*. 30:215-18.

Prasad N K, Bhagat R K and Singh A P.1986. Studies on forage and food based cropping sequences. *Indian J. Agronomy* **31**: 384-86.

Prasad N K, Bhagat R K and Singh A P. 1988. Influence of sowing dates and cutting management on forage production in oats genotypes. *Indian J. of Agronomy* **33**: 372-74.

Prasad N K, Bhagat R K and Singh A P. 1984. Studies on intra and inter row spacing in Subabool (*Leucaena leucocephala). Indian J. of Agronomy* **30**: 113-15

Prasad N K, Bhagat R K and Singh A P. 1985. Comparative production potential of berseem and lucerne under limed and unlimed conditions in oxisol of Chotanagpur plateau. *Indian J. of Agronomy* **30**: 167-71.

Prasad N K, Bhagat R K and Singh A P. 1989. Micronutrients response to Lucerne cultivation in acid soils of Bihar. *Proc. Bihar Acad. Agril. Sci.* **38**; 12-14.

Prasad, N K; Bhagat, R K and Singh, A P. 1990. Response of boron and molybdenum on Lucerne (*Medicago sativa*) forage production. *J. of Res.* BAU. **2**: 11-14.

Prasad, N K; Bhagat R K and Singh A P.1992. Production of hybrid Napier intercropping with cowpea and berseem. *J. of Res. BAU.* **4**: 66-69.

Rai S D, Arora K N and Verma M L.1076. Effect of sowing dates, seed rates and cutting management on the forage yield and nutritive value of oats. *Indian J. Agronomy* **21**:7-10.

Richter Ch, and Marschner H.1973. Umtausch von Kalium in verschiedenen Wurzelzonen von Maiskeimpflanzen. *Z. Pflanzenphysiol* **71**:95-100.

Shankar Vinod (1978) Some effects of burning of tropical grasslands with special reference to their improvement. *Forage Research* **4**: 137-42.

Sekhon G S and Puri D N. 1986. The input-output balance of plant nutrients in some intensive cropping system in India. *Pot. Rev.* **6**: 52-9.

Sharma S K, Ahuja L D, Yadava R P S and Verma C M (1980) Changes in Botanical Composition in the Long Term Seasonal Grazing Paddocks of a desert Rangeland. *Forage Research* **6**: 7-14.

Singh A P and Prasad N K. 1988. Studied on grass-legume association under rainfed conditions of Chotanagpur plateau. *International Rangeland Congress* **2**: 372-74.

Singh A P, Bhagat R K and Prasad N K .1982. Studies on optimum irrigation for oats seed production in Chotanagpur Plateau. *Indian J. of Agronomy* **27**: 202-06

Singh A P, Prasad N K and Bhagat, R K. 1983. Performance of *sarsoon* varieties with berseem. *RAU J. of Res.* **(40)**: 48-51.

Solntanpour, P N, Adams F. and Bennett, A C. 1974. Soil phosphorus availability as measured by displaced soil solutions Calcium chloride-extractants, dilute-acid extractants and labile phosphorus. *Soil Sci. Soc. Am. Proc.* **38**: 225-28.

Taye Bayable, Solomon M and Prasad N K. 2007. Effects of cutting dates on nutritive value of Napier (*P. purpureum*) grass planted sole and in association with Desmodium (*D. intortum*) or Lablab (*L. purpureus*). *Livestock Research for Rularl Development.* **19** (1): 1-12.

Technical Bulletin.1977. CSIRO, Division of Crops and Pasture QLd. Australia.

Trewarth, G. T.1954-68. An introduction to climate, Mc Graw-Hill; New York.

Troll, C.1965. Seasonal Climate of the earth. In E. Rodenwaldh and H. J.Justaz (eds.) World Map of Climatology. Springer- Verlag: New York.

Ullrich W R .1972. DerEinfluB von CO_2 and pHauf die 32p-Markierung von A\Polyphosphaten and organischen Phosphaten bei *Ankistrodesmus braunii* im Licht. Planta **102**:37-54.

U S D A. 1970. Rangeland Cover Types of the United States By: Thomas N Shift, ed. 1994.

Vallentine J F and Sims. 1980. Range Development and Improvement.By: Vallentine J FAcad. Press 3rd ed. June, 1989.

Whyte R O.1964. The Grassland and Fodder Researches of India, ICAR Sci. Monograph No.22.

Willy, R W. 1979. Intercropping to important research needs. I. Competition advantage. *Field Crop Abstracts* **31**:1-10.

Yadava, R B R, Patil, B D and Srinath, P R (1978) Effect of growth regulators on leaf growth, photosynthetic pigments and seed yield of berseem *(T. alexandrinum) Forage Research* **4**: 121-25.

Subject Index

A

Acasia torttilis, 102
Aggressivity, 150
Alpine, 113
Andropojon gayanus, 41
Animal unit, 136
Annuals, 5
Avena sativa, 75

B

Biological competition,150
Brachiaria sps., 42,44
Burning 146

C

C3/C4, 11, 13
CAM, 12
Carrying capacity, 4
CEC, 9, 162,
Cenchrus ciliaris,51
Centrosema sps., 70
Chapparal,121
Chloris gayana, 54
Coix, 38,
CIAT, 58
Colombia, 58
Competitive ratio, 150
Crowding coefficient, 151

Cyamopsis, 61

D

Deferred grazing, 136
Deferred rotational,157
Desert 112
Dichanthium -cenctom - ehyonwous 115

E

Euchalena maxicana , 28

F

Faris banding, 14
Fencing, 148
Farming system, 1
Fodder, 3
Forage, 3
Forage acre, 3
Forage-acre -factor, 4
Forage crop sequences, 152
Forage-food crop sequences,153
Forage-use-factor, 4
Forage value, 4
Forage preservation,123
Forage; food crop systems, 97

G

Grassland, 4
Grazing capacity, 135
Grazing management, 135

H

Hay, 123 HCN,19,24

*Heteropogon contortus,*5 5

Hohenheim system, 137

L

LER, 150

Ley farming, 138

M

Macro-nutrients, 155

Micro-nutrients, 155

Macroptilliunm atropurpureum, 69

Medicage sativa, 90

Monetary advantage, 152

N

Nitrogen cycle, 151

Nutrient concentration in soils, 157

Nutrient in forages, 159

O

Optimization of nutrients in forages, 101

P

Perrisetum glaucum, 25

Panicum maximum, 46

Panicum antidotale, 49

P. pedicellatum, 31

P. perpureum, 33

P. polystachyon 39

P. Cladestinum, 83

Phaseolus calcaratus, 62

Phragmites sacchrum, 116

Prairies, 112

Purarin phaseoloides, 72

P. thunbergia, 72

Q

Q, 10, 14

Quantitative-clinax approach, 145

R

Range management, 141

Reconnaissance, 4

Rotational grazing. 135

Relative-Net Return, 152

S

Savannah,111

Seral., 112

Sehima-Dichanthium, 113

Seral, 4

Sesbania sesban, 101

Setaia spps. 4

Silage, 126

Sorghum bicolor, 17

Steppes, 112

Stocking rate, 135

Stripgraging, 137

Stylosanthes sps., 63, 66

Succession theory, 105

T

Temperate and alpine, 11

Temperate forage, 7

Themeda- ar undinel/a, 116

Trifolium spps., *85*

Tropical forages, 6

Tree phenology, 107

V

Vigna umbellata, 62

Vigna unguiculata, 58

Y

Yarling unit, 136

Z

Zea sps., 27

Zea mays, 29

www.ingramcontent.com/pod-product-compliance
Lightning Source LLC
Chambersburg PA
CBHW021434180326
41458CB00001B/276